Chemically Modified Bodies

Matthew Hall • Sarah Grogan • Brendan Gough
Editors

Chemically Modified Bodies

The Use of Diverse Substances for Appearance Enhancement

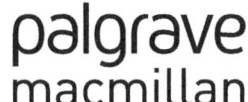

Editors
Matthew Hall
University of Derby
Derby, United Kingdom

Brendan Gough
Leeds Beckett University
Leeds, United Kingdom

Sarah Grogan
Manchester Metropolitan University
Manchester, United Kingdom

ISBN 978-1-137-53534-4   ISBN 978-1-137-53535-1 (eBook)
DOI 10.1057/978-1-137-53535-1

Library of Congress Control Number: 2016937743

© The Editor(s) (if applicable) and The Author(s) 2016
The author(s) has/have asserted their right(s) to be identified as the author(s) of this work in accordance with the Copyright, Designs and Patents Act 1988.
This work is subject to copyright. All rights are solely and exclusively licensed by the Publisher, whether the whole or part of the material is concerned, specifically the rights of translation, reprinting, reuse of illustrations, recitation, broadcasting, reproduction on microfilms or in any other physical way, and transmission or information storage and retrieval, electronic adaptation, computer software, or by similar or dissimilar methodology now known or hereafter developed.
The use of general descriptive names, registered names, trademarks, service marks, etc. in this publication does not imply, even in the absence of a specific statement, that such names are exempt from the relevant protective laws and regulations and therefore free for general use.
The publisher, the authors and the editors are safe to assume that the advice and information in this book are believed to be true and accurate at the date of publication. Neither the publisher nor the authors or the editors give a warranty, express or implied, with respect to the material contained herein or for any errors or omissions that may have been made.

Cover image © Mark Hall
Cover design by Oscar Spigolon

Printed on acid-free paper

This Palgrave Macmillan imprint is published by Springer Nature
The registered company is Macmillan Publishers Ltd. London

Acknowledgments

Editing a collection of divergent research which actively evaluates the emergence of, and apparent increasing use of, non-prescription and prescription drugs for use in changing appearance is not always an easy task. However, this challenge has been made all the more manageable thanks to the flexibility, sensitivity, and collegiate spirit demonstrated by the contributors in this volume. Collectively, we would like to thank them for their contributions and we hope we have done them justice in conveying their voices and their perspectives.

While much of the material is published here for the first time, Chap. 8 has previously appeared in the *Journal of Health Psychology* (Hall et al. 2015). We are grateful to the editors and publishers for permission to reproduce this material here. We would also like to thank Dominic Walker at Palgrave Macmillan, who waited patiently for the manuscript and who saw it through to publication, and the anonymous reviewers for their feedback.

Sarah would also like to thank Naheed Hanif and Dr. Hannah Fawcett for helpful comments on the Smoking and Appearance chapter, and friends and colleagues for consistent support. On a more personal note, Matthew would like to thank his co-editors for their unstinting help and support in putting this volume together; he considers them not only colleagues but also friends. And finally, he would like to say thank you to his family who continually support and enrich his life in many ways.

Matthew Hall
Sarah Grogan
Brendan Gough
November 2015

Contents

1 **Introduction** 1
 Sarah Grogan, Matthew Hall, and Brendan Gough

Part I Background 11

2 **Use of Supplements and Drugs to Change Body Image and Appearance Among Boys and Male Adolescents** 13
 Lina A. Ricciardelli and Robert J. Williams

3 **Muscle Dysmorphia and Anabolic-Androgenic Steroid Use** 31
 Dave Smith, Mary Caitlyn Rutty, and Tracy W. Olrich

4 **Use of Drugs to Change Appearance in Girls and Female Adolescents** 51
 Jennifer O'Dea and Renata Leah Cinelli

Part II Non-prescription Substances — 77

5 Caffeine Misuse and Weight Loss — 79
Carla E. Ramacciotti, Elisabetta Coli, and Annalisa Burgalassi

6 Body Image, Enhancement, and Health in the Advertising of Sports and Nutritional Supplements — 93
Simon Outram

7 Smoking and Appearance — 111
Sarah Grogan

8 Bodybuilders' Accounts of Synthol Use: The Construction of Lay Expertise — 127
Matthew Hall, Sarah Grogan, and Brendan Gough

Part III Prescription Substances — 147

9 Non-Medical Use of ADHD Stimulants for Appetite Suppression and Weight Loss — 149
Amy J. Jeffers and Eric G. Benotsch

10 Commonly Prescribed Oral Anti-Obesity Medication and Alternative Anorectics — 173
Julien S. Baker, Bruce Davies, and Michael R. Graham

11 Peptide Hormones, Metformin and New-Wave Practices and Research Therapies — 201
Michael R. Graham, Julien S. Baker, and Bruce Davies

Afterword: Toward an Inclusive, Multi-Disciplinary Approach to Understanding Substance Use for Appearance Purposes 231
Brendan Gough, Sarah Grogan, and Matthew Hall

Index 235

Notes on Contributors

Julien S. Baker, PhD, DSc is a professor holding fellowships with important and relevant professional organizations, which include: Fellow of the Royal Society of Medicine (FRSM), Fellow of Human Biology Association (FHB), Fellow of the Institute of Biology (FIBiol), Fellow of the Institute of Clinical Research (FICR), and member of the Society for the Study of Biology (SSOB). Professor Baker is also a chartered biologist (CBiol) and chartered scientist (CSci). He is also a member of the Institute for Clinical Research, and a member of both the Physiological Society of Great Britain and the American Physiological Society. He also has membership with the Federation of American Societies for Experimental Biology (FASEB). Professor Baker has published 255 full papers in peer-reviewed journals, published over 290 peer-reviewed abstracts, provided 69 invited key-note presentations, presented at 91 prestigious international conferences, contributed to 19 academic book chapters, written 2 books in partnership, and published 13 invited full papers. His key research areas include high-intensity exercise, immune function, hormonal control, the triglyceride phenotype and obesity, the role of visceral adiposity in cardiovascular disease in children and ethnic minorities, oxidative stress and muscle damage, steroid abuse, and exercise biochemistry.

Eric G. Benotsch, PhD is an Associate Professor of Psychology and director of the health psychology doctoral training program at Virginia Commonwealth University. His research focuses on the use of illicit drugs, misuse of prescription drugs, and HIV prevention.

Annalisa Burgalassi, MD is working as a psychiatrist in the field of mental illness and substances use disorder. Her research at Pisa University focuses on eating disorders.

Renata Leah Cinelli, PhD is a lecturer in Health and Physical Education at Australian Catholic University. Her research focuses on body image, health, and physical activity among adolescent and adult women, with a particular interest in Indigenous Australian women.

Elisabetta Coli, MD practices as a psychiatrist for the Italian National Health Service and continues her research activity at the University of Pisa in the field of eating disorders and obesity, focusing on negative self-esteem as a dimensional perspective pertaining to the spectrum of disturbed eating behaviors.

Bruce Davies, PhD is an emeritus professor in the Faculty of Computing Engineering and Science at the University of South Wales. He has two books and over two hundred book chapters, journal publications, and abstracts to his credit. He is a Fellow of the American College of Medicine, Science and Sport, and a former executive director of the British Olympic medical centre and American Medical International's UK health screening program.

Brendan Gough, PhD is Professor of Social Psychology and qualitative researcher interested in men and masculinities. Now based at Leeds Beckett University, he has published many papers on gender identities and relations, mostly in the context of health, lifestyles, and well-being. Prof. Gough is co-founder and co-editor of the journal *Qualitative Research in Psychology*; he edits the Critical Psychology section of the journal *Social & Personality Psychology Compass*, and is associate editor for the journal *Psychology of Men and Masculinity*. He has co-authored/edited three books in the areas of critical social psychology, reflexivity in qualitative research, and men's health. Recently, he has put together a five-volume *Major Work on Qualitative Research in Psychology* (Sage) and is currently preparing a new *Handbook of Critical Social Psychology* (Palgrave Macmillan) as editor.

Michael R. Graham, PhD has over 30 years of experience in industry, education, research, management and consultancy. He is a visiting professor at the Ningbo University in China. He has more than 50 first-author publications in the area of endocrinology and anti-doping in sport. He is a Fellow of the Royal Society of Medicine and a Chartered Forensic Scientist.

Sarah Grogan, PhD is Professor of Psychology Health and Well-being at Manchester Metropolitan University. Her research focuses on understanding the impact of body image on health-related behaviors such as smoking and anabolic steroid use, and the impact of aging on body image.

Notes on Contributors   xiii

Matthew Hall, PhD is an associate academic at the University of Derby. He is interested in and has published papers on understanding the impacts of multiple and shifting identities and in particular those of gender and sexuality. His current interests also include body modifications and online gender and sexual violence.

Amy J. Jeffers, MS is a doctoral candidate in the Health Psychology program at Virginia Commonwealth University. Her research focuses on substance use and eating disorders/obesity. Specifically, she is interested in the intersection of these topics and how individuals use substances for weight management.

Jennifer O'Dea, MPH, PhD is Professor of Health and Nutrition Education at the University of Sydney. Her research focuses on weight-related health issues in children and adolescents, including body image, self-esteem development, childhood obesity, and the evaluation of school-based health promotion interventions.

Tracy W. Olrich, PhD is a professor in the Department of Physical Education and Sport at Central Michigan University. Dr. Olrich has studied and researched the topic of performance-enhancing substance use in athletics and society for over 25 years. He has several publications on this topic and has made presentations to scholarly, athletic, legislative, and lay communities concerning the issue.

Simon Outram, PhD is a research fellow at the Institute of Sport, Exercise & Active Living (ISEAL), Victoria University, Melbourne. He has a multi-disciplinary background including social anthropology, science and technology studies, and bioethics. In his current position at ISEAL, Simon is exploring the social, ethical, and policy implications and status of supplement use in sport. His research also concerns the conceptualization of performance enhancement, naturalness, and fairness within sport, especially in relation to the prohibition of some substances within sport. He has also conducted research into the governance of anti-doping in sport.

Carla E. Ramacciotti, MD is a professor at Pisa University. Her research focuses on clinics and treatment of eating disorders, and more recently also on ortorexia nervosa and obesity.

Lina A. Ricciardelli, PhD is a professor in the School of Psychology at Deakin University, Australia. Her research focuses on sociocultural factors and the development of body image and other health risk behaviors among children, adolescents, and adults. These have included gender-role stereotypes, sport, the media, peers, the family, and culture.

Mary Caitlyn Rutty, BS (Psychol), ACSM is a Research Assistant at Central Michigan University aiding in teaching and research involving performance-enhancing drugs, and psychosocial aspects of sport in the Department of Physical Education and Sport.

Dave Smith, PhD is Senior Lecturer in Sport Psychology at Manchester Metropolitan University. His research explores psychological issues in bodybuilding and strength training, including exercise dependence, muscle dysmorphia and drug use, and effects of low back pain therapies.

Robert J. Williams, PhD is currently researching comparative perspectives on the embodiment of consciousness as conceptualized in phenomenological and cognitive psychology "as it reaches beyond the New Age," in the School of Letters, Arts and Media, University of Sydney. His earlier research focused on substance use, self-management, and gender-role stereotypes.

List of Figures

Fig. 10.1	Orlistat (Xenical)	179
Fig. 10.2	Ephedrine	181
Fig. 10.3	(a) Triiodothyronine (T_3) (b) Tetraiodothyronine (T_4)	184
Fig. 10.4	Thyroid system	185
Fig. 10.5	Clenbuterol	187
Fig. 10.6	Sibutramine	189
Fig. 11.1	The GH–IGF axis and regulation of GH and IGF-I synthesis and secretion	208
Fig. 11.2	Human growth hormone in its correct 22-kD-hGH form	214
Fig. 11.3	Insulin-like growth factor (IGF-I)	220

List of Tables

Table 4.1	Drug use for weight control in male and female Australian adolescents of low, middle, and high socioeconomic status in 2012	59
Table 4.2	Smoking for weight loss in male and female Australian adolescents of low, middle, and high socioeconomic status in 2012	61
Table 10.1	The international classification of adult underweight, overweight, and obesity values according to BMI	176
Table 10.2	Drugs commonly used to treat obesity in the UK and USA	177

1

Introduction

Sarah Grogan, Matthew Hall, and Brendan Gough

Body Image and Drug Use

All chapters in this book focus on aspects of body image. In recent years, there has been a noticeable increase in academic and popular interest in psychological factors related to body image and appearance concern (Cash 2012). Researchers have also become increasingly interested in people's experiences of embodiment and drug use, and the impact of body image and appearance on drug use (e.g. Hildebrandt and Alfano 2012; Grogan et al. 2009; McCabe and Ricciardelli 2003; Yager and

---

S. Grogan (✉)
Department of Psychology, Manchester Metropolitan University, 53 Bonsall Street, M15 6GX, Manchester, UK

M. Hall
Associate Academic, University of Derby, Department of Psychology, Kedleston Road, Derby DE22 1GB, UK

B. Gough
School of Social, Psychological and Communication Sciences, Leeds Beckett University, Calverly Building [Rm 919], City Campus, LS1 9HE, Leeds, UK

© The Editor(s) (if applicable) and The Author(s) 2016
M. Hall et al. (eds.), *Chemically Modified Bodies*,
DOI 10.1057/978-1-137-53535-1_1

O'Dea 2014). The significant rise in the use of drugs designed to make men and women more muscular and thinner has inspired researchers to try to understand motivations behind these behaviours, and more general experiences of embodiment that may be impacted by drug use.

The earliest published definition of body image was, "The picture of our own body which we form in our mind, that is to say, the way in which the body appears to ourselves" (Schilder 1950, p. 11). Since 1950, researchers have taken body image to mean many different things, and have moved beyond Schilder's focus on perceptual factors to consider a wide range of issues such as weight satisfaction, size perception accuracy, appearance satisfaction, body satisfaction, appearance evaluation, appearance orientation, body concern, body esteem, body schema, and body percept (Thompson 2012). In an attempt to incorporate the key elements, Grogan (2008) used the definition, "A person's perceptions, thoughts, and feelings about his or her body" (p. 3). This definition can be taken to include psychological concepts such as perception and attitudes towards the body as well as experiences of embodiment. Perceptual body image is usually measured by investigating accuracy of body size estimation relative to actual size. Attitudinal body image is assessed using measures of four components: global subjective satisfaction (evaluation of the body), affect (feelings associated with the body), cognitions (investment in appearance, beliefs about the body), and behaviours (such as avoidance of situations where the body will be exposed). Psychological measures of body image assess one or more of these components (Thompson 2012).

To understand body image fully, it needs to be investigated from a range of psychological viewpoints; we need to look not only at individuals' experiences in relation to their bodies, but also at the cultural settings in which people live and the ways that they make sense of how their bodies look within different kinds of social contexts. This text will present work on links between drug use and body image from a number of perspectives, to try to understand both individual and societal factors relating to body image and drug use. Recent evidence has shown that males and females of all ages use various drugs to try to change the looks of their bodies, usually to find ways to be thinner for women and girls, and slender and muscular for men and boys. Drug use may also be impacted by other kinds of appearance concerns, such as the desire to look young and wrinkle-free (Grogan et al. 2010a), and these issues will also be addressed later in this text.

Drugs to Reduce Weight

In spite of cultural awareness of the need to reduce objectification of women's bodies, there remains significant sociocultural pressure on women to be slender and toned (Frith 2012; Tiggemann and Andrew 2012), and many women of all ages are dissatisfied with aspects of their bodies and most want to be slimmer (Grogan et al. 2013; Tiggemann and McCourt 2013). Men are also under some cultural pressure to be slender as well as muscular, and although most research on men's body image has focused on the desire for larger and more defined muscles (Fawkner 2012; Hale and Smith 2012; McCreary 2012), there is good evidence that most men and adolescent boys desire to look lean as well as muscular (Grogan and Richards 2002; Ricciardelli 2012). Body builders are also increasingly seeking drugs that will reduce body fat in addition to those that will build muscle (Hall et al. 2014; Magkos and Kavouras 2004).

The use of diet pills is a major health issue, linked with anxiety, restlessness, and insomnia, with high and sustained use being linked to increased risk of myocardial infarction and stroke (Calfee and Fadale 2006; Medicinenet.com 2015). The use of caffeine to control weight is an important area of new research, and heavy caffeine use has been implicated in serious health problems in women who use heavy doses to control their weight (Ramacciotti et al. 2016). Prescription substances such as stimulants designed to treat attention deficit disorder also suppress appetite, and there is now some evidence that people are using them for weight loss rather than their intended purpose (Jeffers and Benotsch 2014). Also, substances such as clenbuterol, ephedrine, recombinant human growth hormone, thyroxine, and orlistat can cause serious long-term problems if used for appearance reasons and without medical supervision (Baker et al. 2016). Recently the role of cigarette smoking among young women to control weight has been investigated, and has been found to represent a serious health concern (Grogan 2012). Also, both male and female smokers tend to have lower body satisfaction than never-smokers, and may be concerned about stopping smoking because of the likely impact on their weight after quitting (Grogan et al. 2009, 2010b).

Drugs to Increase Muscularity

Men are under increasing pressure to become more muscular (Hildebrandt and Alfano 2012; Thompson and Cafri 2007), and may resort to drugs to enable them to increase muscularity. The rise in the use of appearance- and performance-enhancing drugs such as anabolic steroids, used by men and some women (Grogan et al. 2006), presents significant health risks, including increased risk of heart attacks and strokes (NHS 2015). These drugs may be particularly common in those with muscle dysmorphia (Hildebrandt and Alfano 2012), although their use is becoming increasingly widespread across broader populations (Kimergård and McVeigh 2014). This has led to serious health concerns about needle use and the health impacts of the anabolic steroids themselves, particularly when taken in heavy doses recommended by some online information sites (Grogan et al. 2006).

Growth hormone is now widely available for non-medicinal use, and can cause health problems if taken, without medical support, by those wanting to produce appearance-related changes (Graham et al. 2016). Substances such as synthol, which are injected into desired muscles in order to make those muscles appear bigger, are also widely available on the Internet (Hall et al. 2015) and may carry a wide range of health risks including destroying the injected muscle (Ghandourah et al. 2012).

Summary of Book Content

In this book we investigate both prescription and non-prescription drugs, focusing on their impact on appearance, and the psychological and health-related factors linked with their use. In the first section, we focus on some of the differential aspects of drug use within males and females, and also review use of appearance-related drugs by those with body dysmorphic disorder. Chapter 2 investigates use of drugs to change appearance in boys and male adolescents, focusing on links between drug use and the desire to become more muscular, gain body size and weight, and increase body strength. Links are made with use of appearance- and performance-enhancing drugs such as anabolic-androgenic steroids, food supplements, creatine, ephedrine, and adrenal hormones. This is followed by a consideration of body dysmorphic disorder in Chap. 3, investigating links between muscle dysmorphia and drug use, including use of anabolic steroids and treatment issues. Chapter 4 will consider use of drugs to change appearance in girls and female adolescents, focusing in particular on concerns about overweight and the desire to be more slender.

The second section focuses on non-prescription substances, looking first at use of caffeine as a slimming aid. Chapter 5 will focus on appearance-related motivations for caffeine use, poorer body image, and body weight anxieties, as well as considering health impacts of heavy use. Chapter 6 will explore the demand for dietary supplements in relation to physical appearance, linked to cultural intolerance of imperfections in health and appearance. Chapter 7 focusses on links between cigarette smoking and weight concern, and also looks at how appearance concerns related to youthful-looking skin might be used in positive ways to enable smokers to quit. Chapter 8 investigates use of the injectable oil known as synthol, used by bodybuilders to enhance the size of muscle. There is evidence that this drug appears to have become increasingly popular in mainstream bodybuilding and it is widely available on the Internet.

The third section investigates use of prescription substances, and starts with a consideration of the use of stimulants used to treat attention deficit disorder as appetite suppressants by those wanting to lose weight in Chap. 9. Chapter 10 focusses on use of drugs to increase metabolic rate such as ephedrine, and prevent fat absorption, such as orlistat. Possible negative health impacts if these drugs are taken within medical support are considered. Chapter 11 considers the impact of insulin, growth hormone, and metformin, all available through the Internet and marketed as ways to improve appearance. Possible positive and negative impacts are considered. In the Afterword, we consider further directions for other researchers and future research areas.

Conclusions

Clearly there are important links between body image and drug use. This text will attempt to produce a summary of current knowledge and research relating drug (mis)use to appearance concern and body image, exploring drug use from a variety of psychosocial perspectives, and drawing on a range of methodologies. It is important to gain information from studies where people are interviewed about reasons for drug use or where already-existing data from Internet discussion boards are examined, to help in understanding how people make sense of their drug use within a context of (often considerable) health risks. It is also crucial to understand directional links between body image and drug use, so experimental and longitudinal studies where drug use and body image are examined in controlled ways will also be reviewed. Presenting a full picture of links between appearance concerns and use of drugs to change appearance will enable us to identify clear implications for health promotion interventions designed to prevent or reduce drug (mis)use. Therefore, this book is likely to be of interest to a range of scholars, practitioners, support groups, policymakers, media, and students from fields as diverse as medicine, pharmacology, psychology and psychiatry, gender studies, nutrition and sociology who are interested in issues such as substance (ab)use, addictions, gender identity, body image, and some of the complex links between drug use and body image.

References

Baker, J. S., Davies, B., & Graham, M. R. (2016). Commonly prescribed oral anti-obesity medication and alternative anorectics. In M. Hall, S. Grogan, & B. Gough (Eds.), *Chemically modified bodies*. London: Palgrave Macmillan.

Calfee, R., & Fadale, F. (2006). Popular ergogenic drugs and supplements in young athletes. Pediatrics, 117, 577–589.

Cash, T. (2012). Preface. In T. F. Cash (Ed.), *Encyclopedia of body image and human appearance* (pp. xix–xxx). London: Elsevier.

Fawkner, H. J. (2012). Body image development—Adult men. In T. Cash (Ed.), *Encyclopedia of body image and human appearance* (pp. 194–201). London: Elsevier.

Frith, H. (2012). Appearance and society. In N. Rumsey & D. Harcourt (Eds.), *The Oxford handbook of the psychology of appearance* (pp. 10–23). Oxford: Oxford University Press.

Ghandourah, S., Hofer, M. J., Kiebling, A., El-Zayat, B., & Dietmar Schofar, M. (2012). Painful muscle fibrosis following synthol injections in a bodybuilder: A case report. *Journal of Medical Case Reports, 6*, 248.

Graham, M. R., Baker, J. S., & Davies, B. (2016). Peptide hormones, metformin and new-wave practices and research therapies. In M. Hall, S. Grogan, & B. Gough (Eds.), *Chemically modified bodies*. London: Palgrave Macmillan.

Grogan, S. (2008). *Body image: Understanding body dissatisfaction in men, women and children* (2nd ed.). London: Routledge.

Grogan, S. (2012). Smoking and body image. In T. Cash (Ed.), *Encyclopedia of body image and human appearance* (pp. 745–750). London: Elsevier.

Grogan, S., & Richards, H. (2002). Body image: Focus groups with boys and men. *Men and Masculinities, 4*, 219–232.

Grogan, S., Shepherd, S., Evans, R., Wright, S., & Hunter, G. (2006). Body builders experiences of anabolic steroid use: In-depth interviews with men and women body builders. *Psychology and Health, 11*, 845–856.

Grogan, S., Fry, G., Gough, B., & Conner, M. (2009). Smoking to stay thin or giving up to save face. Young men and women talk about appearance concerns and smoking. *British Journal of Health Psychology, 14*, 175–186.

Grogan, S., Flett, K., Clark-Carter, D., Gough, B., Davey, R., Richardson, D., et al. (2010a). Women smokers' experiences of an age-appearance anti-smoking intervention: A qualitative study. *British Journal of Health Psychology, 16*, 675–689.

Grogan, S., Hartley, L., Fry, G., Conner, M., & Gough, B. (2010b). Appearance concerns and smoking in young men and women: Going beyond weight control. *Drugs: Education, Prevention and Policy, 17*, 261–269.

Grogan, S., Gill, S., Brownbridge, K., Kilgariff, S., & Whalley, A. (2013). Dress fit and body image: A thematic analysis of women's accounts during and after trying on dresses. *Body Image, 10*, 380–388.

Hale, B. D., & Smith, D. (2012). Bodybuilding. In T. Cash (ed.), *Encyclopedia of body image and human appearance* (pp. 66–74). London: Elsevier.

Hall, M., Grogan, S., & Gough, B. (2014). "It is safe to use if you are healthy": A discursive analysis of men's online accounts of ephedrine use. *Psychology and Health*. doi:10.1080/08870446.2014.994632.

Hall, M., Grogan, S., & Gough, B. (2015). Bodybuilders' accounts of synthol use: The construction of lay expertise. *Journal of Health Psychology*. doi:10.1177/1359105314568579.

Hildebrandt, T., & Alfano, L. (2012). Drug use, appearance- and performance-enhancing. In T. Cash (Ed.), *Encyclopedia of body image and human appearance* (pp. 392–398). London: Elsevier.

Jeffers, A., & Benotsch, E. G. (2014). Non-medical use of prescription stimulants for weight loss, disordered eating, and body image. *Eating Behaviors, 15*, 3.

Kimergård, A., & McVeigh, J. (2014). Variability and dilemmas in harm reduction for anabolic steroid users in the UK: A multi-area interview study. *Harm Reduction Journal, 11*, 19.

Magkos, F., & Kavouras, S. A. (2004). Caffeine and ephedrine. *Sports Medicine., 34*, 871–889.

McCabe, M. P., & Ricciardelli, L. A. (2003). Body image and strategies to lose weight and increase muscle among boys and girls. *Health Psychology, 22*, 39–46.

McCreary, D. R. (2012). Muscularity and body image. In T. Cash (Ed.), *Encyclopedia of body image and human appearance* (pp. 561–567). London: Elsevier.

Medicinenet.com. (2015). *Ephedrine-oral*. Accessed April 3, 2015, from http://www.medicinenet.com/ephedrine-oral/article.htm

National Health Service. (2015). *Anabolic steroid misuse*. Accessed March 24, 2015, from http://www.nhs.uk/conditions/anabolic-steroid-abuse/Pages/Introduction.aspx

Ramacciotti, C. E., Coli, E., & Burgalassi, A. (2016). Caffeine misuse and weight loss. In M. Hall, S. Grogan, & B. Gough (Eds.), *Chemically modified bodies*. London: Palgrave Macmillan.

Ricciardelli, L. A. (2012). Body image development—Adolescent boys. In T. Cash (Ed.), *Encyclopedia of body image and human appearance* (pp. 180–187). London: Elsevier.

Schilder, P. (1950). *The image and appearance of the human body*. New York: International Universities Press.

Thompson, J. K. (2012). Measurement of body image in adolescence and adulthood. In T. Cash (Ed.), *Encyclopedia of body image and human appearance* (pp. 512–521). London: Elsevier.

Thompson, J. K., & Cafri, G. (Eds.) (2007). *The muscular ideal*. Washington, DC: APA.

Tiggemann, M., & Andrew, R. (2012). Clothing choices, weight, and trait self-objectification. *Body Image, 9*, 409–412.

Tiggemann, M., & McCourt, A. (2013). Body appreciation in adult women: Relationships with age and body satisfaction. *Body Image, 10*, 624–627.

Yager, Z., & O'Dea, J. A. (2014). Relationships between body image, nutritional supplement use, and attitudes towards doping in sport among adolescent boys: Implications for prevention programs. *Journal of the International Society of Sports Nutrition, 11*, 13.

Part I

Background

2

Use of Supplements and Drugs to Change Body Image and Appearance Among Boys and Male Adolescents

Lina A. Ricciardelli and Robert J. Williams

Background

It is estimated that between 40 and 70 % of adolescent boys are dissatisfied with some aspect of their body image (e.g. Almeida et al. 2012; Huenemann et al. 1966; Lawler and Nixon 2011; Lerner 1972; McCabe and Ricciardelli 2004a; Ricciardelli et al. 2006). This may include dissatisfaction with body size and weight, muscularity, and/or height; and dissatisfaction with specific body parts such as biceps, shoulders, and chest. It also includes dissatisfaction with more functional aspects of one's body which are often required for playing sports. These include speed, strength, fitness, stamina, endurance, and physical co-ordination. While most researchers have primarily studied adolescent males, studies have also shown that as many as 50 % of preadolescent boys, aged as

L.A. Ricciardelli (✉)
School of Psychology, Deakin University, Burwood Highway, 221, 3125 Burwood, VIC, Australia

R.J. Williams
School of Letters, Arts and Media, University of Sydney, Carr Street, 28/58, 2034 Coogee, NSW, Australia

© The Editor(s) (if applicable) and The Author(s) 2016
M. Hall et al. (eds.), *Chemically Modified Bodies*,
DOI 10.1057/978-1-137-53535-1_2

young as 8 years old, display similar body image concerns as adolescent boys. As with adolescent males, younger boys are preoccupied with both leanness and muscularity (e.g. Dunn et al. 2010; Grogan and Richards 2002; Tatangelo and Ricciardelli 2013), and place great importance on obtaining a fit body which is highly desired for strengthening sporting performance.

Given the array of body image concerns displayed by boys, it is not surprising that many boys have been found to use a range of body-change strategies in order to modify and improve their body image and appearance concerns. The main body-change strategies used by boys include increasing exercise and modifying eating patterns (Eisenberg et al. 2012; Ricciardelli and McCabe 2004; Smolak et al. 2005). However, many boys use a range of supplements and substances often referred to as appearance- and performance-enhancing drugs (APEDs; Hildebrandt et al. 2012). Given that their use is usually associated with body image concerns, these supplements and drugs have also been referred to as 'body image drugs' (Kanayama et al. 2012). These include steroids, which are viewed as highly desirable, as they permit users to achieve marked increases in muscularity and decreases in body fat, which are well beyond the limits attainable by natural means (Kanayama et al. 2012). In addition, steroids are often used in combination with other drugs to gain muscle or lose body fat, which include human growth hormones, thyroid hormones, insulin, clenbuterol, and ephedrine (Kanayama et al. 2012). Moreover, APEDs include stimulants, and diet pills, powders, or liquids that can be used to reduce body weight/composition (Thorlton et al. 2012).

In this chapter, we first review the range and prevalence of APEDs among adolescent boys. In addition, we review the factors that have been shown to increase the risk that boys use APEDs, and we highlight the areas that require more extensive research.

Types of Supplements and Drugs, and Prevalence

Many boys use muscle-building supplements and drugs which include steroids, steroid precursors, and nutritional supplements (Hildebrandt et al. 2012). Estimates for the number of adolescent boys who have ever used steroids range from 1.2 % to 12 % (Harmer 2010; Ricciardelli and McCabe 2004; Thorlton et al. 2012; van den Berg et al. 2007). In a recent representative sample of secondary high school students in Australia, the lifetime use of steroids was found to be 2.4 % among 12- to 17-year-olds (Dunn and White 2011). More specifically, 1.8 % had used steroids in the last year and 1.0 % had used steroids in the last month. In another recent study conducted in the USA, the lifetime use of steroids among adolescents (mean age 14.4 years) was found to be 5.9 %, with 0.8 % who reported using steroids frequently (Eisenberg et al. 2012). More precisely, one study found that among adolescents who used steroids, 18 % reported monthly use, 18 % reported weekly use, and 10 % reported daily use (van den Berg et al. 2007).

Steroid precursors include creatine, ephedrine, adrenal hormones, amino acids, and prohormones (Field et al. 2005; Hildebrandt et al. 2012). It is estimated that between 1.5 % and 23 % of adolescent boys have used these substances in their lifetime. In addition, it is estimated that these steroid precursors are used frequently by 2.4 % of boys (Eisenberg et al. 2012). Other supplements also used by boys to increase muscle size and tone are protein powders and bars, sport drinks such as Gatorade and Powerade; vitamins or minerals; and energy drinks such as Red Bull (Yager and O'Dea 2014). Estimates for these more easily accessible supplements range from 33 % to 49.9 % (Smolak et al. 2005; Yager and O'Dea 2014); with 6.3 % of adolescents reporting the use of these supplements regularly (Eisenberg et al. 2012). Although most studies have been conducted with adolescent males, in one study we conducted with preadolescent boys, we found that the use of food supplements to increase muscles was similar to that found among this younger age group: 41.9 % of boys aged between 8 and 11 years frequently reported eating "special foods" (e.g. protein powders) to increase their muscles (Ricciardelli et al. 2003).

In addition to muscle-building supplements, adolescents use a range of other supplements and drugs for controlling and/or modifying their weight (Thorlton et al. 2012). These include tobacco, diet pills, diuretics and laxatives, which are usually used for weight loss (Hildebrandt et al. 2012; Thorlton et al. 2012). It is estimated that between 1 % to 5.6 % of boys smoke cigarettes to lose weight; 0.1 % to 4.7 % of boys use diet pills; and 0.1 % to 1.6 % of boys use laxatives (e.g., Field et al. 1999;

Krowchuck et al. 1998; López-Guimeró et al. 2013; Neumark-Sztainer et al. 1999; Ross and Ivis 1999; Stephen et al. 2014; Thorlton et al. 2012; Whitaker et al. 1989; Vander Wal 2011). In addition to tobacco, adolescents have also been found to use a range of other stimulants for weight loss. These include methamphetamines such as speed, crystal, crank or ice, which have been found to be used by 4.9 % of adolescent boys (Thorlton et al. 2012).

Stimulants such as caffeine and energy drinks have also been reported to be used by adolescents for weight loss (Jeffers et al. 2014). Caffeine can act as an appetite suppressant and it is also known for its diuretic purposes (Jeffers et al. 2014). Energy drinks include both caffeine and another stimulant, bitter orange, which is also used as weight management product, and both substances are frequently marketed as stimulating weight loss (Jeffers et al. 2014). In addition, adolescents have been found to misuse prescription drugs as stimulants for weight loss. These include medications to treat attention deficit hyperactivity disorder, such as Adderall and Ritalin (Jeffers and Benotsch 2014). However, we have only prevalence data on the use of caffeine and energy drinks, and the misuse of prescription drugs for the purpose of weight loss among adults. In one study, 56.9 % of adults who were trying to lose weight reported using energy drinks (Jeffers et al. 2014). In another study, the misuse of prescription drugs for weight loss was found to be 6.7 % among college males (Jeffers and Benotsch 2014). Prevalence data for adolescents on these substances is now needed.

Risk Factors

A range of risk factors have been found to be associated with the use of APEDs among boys and adolescent males. Many of these factors are similar to those found to be associated with disordered eating and other strategies that males use to attain a more lean and muscular body size (Ricciardelli and McCabe 2004). These include psychosocial factors such as body image and appearance concerns, sociocultural pressures, the sporting environment, and negative affect and self-esteem; and biological factors such as age, body mass index (BMI), and puberty. Boys and adolescent males experience pressures from all directions. There are sociocultural pressures which include extensive messages from a range of media (TV, magazines, films, and the Internet) that consistently promote the muscular ideal body image for males. This is also a time when boys' bodies are developing, and before puberty many boys may feel that their bodies are inadequate and are a long way from reaching the muscular ideal. Boys also receive many pressures to perform well at sports in order to attain status and popularity, as this is also an important context for boys as they can provide a masculine display of muscularity and strength. In addition, given that adolescence is a time of increased experimentation and risk taking, adolescents with higher body image and appearance concerns are especially vulnerable to health-risk behaviours. Thus, the use of APEDs among adolescent males can be viewed as one of the high health-risk behaviours.

Body image and appearance concerns. It is well established that adolescent boys with more body image and appearance concerns are more likely to use APEDs (Bahrke et al. 2000). In addition, initiation of steroid use for enhanced appearance or body image, and increase in size and/or strength is reported to be the main underlying motivation (Sagoe et al. 2014). For example, in one early study, boys who reported frequently thinking about wanting more defined muscles and those wanting to gain weight were more likely to use products to improve appearance, muscle mass, or strength (Field et al. 2005). These products included protein powders or shakes, creatine, amino acids, growth hormones, or steroids. Similarly, in a more recent survey of adolescent males, 9.2 % of 16–22-year-olds who were very concerned with muscularity reported using a variety of substances, including creatine and dehydroepiandrosterone supplements, growth hormone derivatives, and anabolic steroids to improve physical appearance or to help gain weight, strength, or muscle mass (Field et al. 2014).

Body image concerns during adolescence have also been found to retrospectively predict lifetime steroid use among experienced weight lifters (Pope et al. 2012). Specifically, this included measures tapping adolescent body image with a focus on muscularity, self-reported adolescent physical attractiveness, and athleticism from the Adolescent Experience

Questionnaire designed by authors; and scores on the muscle dysmorphia version of the Yale-Brown Obsessive Compulsive Scale.

Body mass index and weight status. There is some evidence that both underweight and overweight adolescents have greater body image concerns in comparison to adolescent males who are in the normal weight range (McCabe and Ricciardelli 2004a). Thus, both underweight and overweight adolescents may be at greater risk of using APEDs. However, only a few studies have examined the relationship between BMI and/or weight status in relation to the use of APEDs. Most studies have not included an assessment of BMI (e.g. Dunn and White 2011; Harrison and Bond 2007; Smolak et al. 2005); and BMI was also not considered in two large reviews of the literature (Bahrke et al. 2000; Sagoe et al. 2014). In an early study, low BMI was found to be weakly associated with the use of steroids and food supplements (Neumark-Sztainer et al. 1999). On the other hand, in a more recent study, overweight and obese adolescent boys were found to be more likely to report muscle-enhancing behaviours (Eisenberg et al. 2012). However, other studies have found no relationship between BMI and the use of APEDs among adolescent males (e.g., Ricciardelli and McCabe 2003; Rodgers et al. 2012; Thorlton et al. 2012). Given the limited number of studies that have examined this relationship, additional studies are clearly needed before clear conclusions can be drawn.

Age and pubertal development. Most studies have shown that the average age adolescents commence using steroids is 15 years. However, boys have also been found to begin using steroids as early as 10 years old (Bahrke et al. 2000). In a recent representative sample of secondary high school students in Australia (Dunn and White 2011), the lifetime use of steroids was found to be more common among 12–15-year-olds (2.6 %) than 16–17-year-olds (1.9 %). This was also the case in an earlier study, which found that students in middle school were more likely to report using steroids than students in high school (Irving et al. 2002). It may be that younger boys are more affected by sociocultural pressures which promote the muscular ideal as they are more out of sync with the societal ideal shape for a man. As boys develop they add muscle and their shoulder width increases, and this moves them closer to the muscular ideal (Ricciardelli and McCabe 2004). In support of this view, late-maturing boys have been found to be more likely to use food supplements to build up their body than early maturing boys, and this predicted an increased use of other strategies to increase their muscle size (McCabe and Ricciardelli 2004b). Additional studies are needed to more fully examine the effects of puberty and how these may moderate and/or mediate other risk factors. For example, late-maturing boys may be more vulnerable to the effects of psychosocial factors, such as sociocultural pressures and negative affect.

Sociocultural pressures. Increasingly boys and men are experiencing greater social pressure to attain a muscular body from the media, and this is viewed as contributing to their body dissatisfaction and other body image concerns. There has been a growing trend for muscular male bodies to be featured in popular magazines, television, and films (e.g. Labre 2005; Leit et al. 2001; Morrison and Halton 2009). For example, magazines that feature images of muscular men, such as *Men's Health* and *Men's Fitness* are commonly dominated by articles that focus on leanness and muscularity. One content analysis showed that 25 % of articles in these magazines focussed on 'burning fat and building muscle', followed by articles that focussed on other aspects of mental or physical health (18 %). This also included advertisements focussed on APEDs (16 %); and leanness or muscularity was the most frequently purported benefit of using the products that were advertised (Labre 2005).

In addition, it has been found that action figures such as *GI Joe* and *Star Wars* figurines have increased in muscularity over time, with major increases in the chest and shoulder measurements (Pope et al. 1999). Current models of these toys far exceed levels of muscularity that are achievable by adult human beings, let alone young boys. Similarly, research that mapped the body dimensions of male characters in the top 150 video games showed that they were significantly and disproportionally larger than the average American male (Martins et al. 2010).

In one study, Field et al. (2005) found a direct relationship between media exposure and the use of APEDs. Specifically, adolescent boys who read men's, teen, fashion, or health and fitness magazines were more likely to use APEDs (Field et al. 2005). In another study, Harrison and Bond (2007) found that exposure to video gaming magazines predicted a significant increase in drive for muscularity one year later among White preadolescent boys (mean age = 8.77 years). Video gaming magazines were selected as these include bulky and beefed-up characters, and drive for muscularity was assessed using McCreary and Sasse's (2000) adapted scale for preadolescent boys, which included items such as, "I eat special foods to make my muscles bigger" and "I drink special shakes to make my muscles bigger".

Additional studies have shown that the sociocultural pressures associated with using APEDs and other strategies to increase muscles extend beyond media influences to also include pressure or comments from family and peers. In one study, media influence, defined as the use of media, which included TV, movies, and magazines to obtain information about body shape; perceived comments from parents (e.g. "Your father made comments or teased you about not being muscular or strong enough"); and peer pressure which assessed boys' perceptions of their friends and classmates' investment in body shape and muscularity (e.g. "How often do your friends and classmates encourage each other to lift weights?") were all found to be significantly higher among adolescents who used food supplements and/or steroids versus those who did not (Smolak et al. 2005). Similarly, in a more recent study Rodgers et al. (2012) found that both perceived pressure to gain muscles and pressure to lose weight from media, family members, and peers, and the internalisation of the ideal body as portrayed by the media predicted adolescents' drive for muscularity. The drive for muscularity was assessed by McCreary and Sasse's (2000) scale and included items such as, "I use protein or energy supplements" and "I think about taking anabolic steroids".

Cultural background. The influence of sociocultural factors has also been studied by examining the use of APEDs in other cultures and/or countries. The use of steroids has been found to be a larger problem in Scandinavia followed by the USA, British Commonwealth countries, Brazil, and the rest of Western Europe (Kanayama et al. 2012). On the other hand, the abuse of steroids is rare in Eastern countries such as China, Korea, and Japan (Kanayama et al. 2012). The greater use of steroids in Western countries is attributed to the high value placed on muscularity in the West which is highlighted by mythical heroes, such as Hercules in Ancient Greece and Thor in mythical traditions of Scandinavia (Kanayama et al. 2012). These have continued to be idealised in modern times with muscular action toys, magazine advertisements, and Hollywood films. The Western muscular historic heroes and Hollywood role models are a contrast to what we see in the East. For example, ancient deities in Japan are fully clothed with no efforts to enhance muscularity, and the teachings of Confucius link masculinity to intellect, refinement, and virtuousness, and not to brawn (Kanayama et al. 2012). Similarly in modern-day China and Japan, one rarely sees images of muscularity. On the contrary, the focus in popular Asian action films is on lean martial artists and not muscle-bound characters (Kanayama et al. 2012).

While the use of steroids among males in Asian countries is very low, Asian boys living in the USA have been found to be more likely to use steroids than Whites (Eisenberg et al. 2012). Moreover, the highest rate of steroid use was reported by Hmong respondents: 14.8 % versus 5.4 % of other adolescent males (Eisenberg et al. 2012). The Hmong are a more recent immigrant group and the researchers argued that they may be bulking up to gain status in a culture that emphases physical appearance. Another study from the USA has also found higher steroid use among Native American adolescents as compared to Whites (van den Berg et al. 2007). Although additional studies are needed to verify the findings, the higher level of steroid use among adolescent males from minority groups in the USA is consistent with the findings of our review which showed that many males from minority groups demonstrated more body image concerns and body-change strategies than Whites (Ricciardelli et al. 2007). We argued that these differences may in part reflect the changing status quo and power relations for males and/or the higher level of social isolation of men in minority groups when compared to the dominant cultural group(s). In particular, men more than women are worse off in a climate of emerging acculturation and modernisation as they may have more to lose than to gain in their social status with changing social structures.

Sport environment and participation. Another important sociocultural sphere of influence for boys is sport. Sport is often pivotal to the lives of boys, as many spend a lot of time playing a range of sports and sport also provides boys with a supportive social environment for developing friendships (Coleman 2011; Ricciardelli et al. 2006; Tatangelo and Ricciardelli 2013). Participation in any kind of sport for boys is related to higher self-esteem (Holland and Andre 1994), and adolescent boys more than girls perceive that the function of sport participation is to increase their social status and peer popularity (White et al. 1998). In addition, the sporting context is the main forum that Western males have for demonstrating the various aspects of masculinity which are closely aligned with the pursuit of muscularity. In our interview study with adolescent boys we found that what boys liked about their bodies and the aspects they wanted to improve were synonymous with the attributes associated with being successful at sport. These included functional aspects of the body such as overall size, height, speed, strength, fitness, and endurance (Ricciardelli et al. 2006).

Sport participation has been reported as a major reason for why adolescent boys use steroids (Bahrke et al. 2000). Steroids are used to increase one's physical size and muscle strength, which are closely related to improved sporting performance. The main sports found to be associated with steroid use among adolescents and adult males are primarily the ones that focus on muscular strength and size-dependent sports of football, wrestling, and track and field events (Bahrke et al. 2000; Field et al. 2005; Ricciardelli and McCabe 2004; Sagoe et al. 2014). However, 30 to 40 % of adolescents use steroids for more individual sporting pursuits which include bodybuilding and/or weightlifting (Bahrke et al. 2000; Field et al. 2005). These and other sports that focus on muscular strength are also referred to as 'power sports' (Ricciardelli and McCabe 2004; Sagoe et al. 2014).

Substance abuse and other risk-taking behaviours. An early hypothesis that was proposed but has not been supported is that adolescents who use steroids would be less likely to use other illicit drugs, as these would jeopardise their health and athletic performance (Bahrke et al. 2000). However, studies have consistently shown that adolescents who use steroids use a range of legal and illicit drugs (Bahrke et al. 2000; Dunn and White 2011). In one study, adolescents who had used steroids were also more likely to have used cigarettes, alcohol, marijuana, and 'other drugs', such as acid, crack, and cocaine (van den Berg et al. 2007). In another study, adolescents who used steroids reported experimenting with other substances, including alcohol, tobacco, cannabis, cocaine, or heroin (Dunn and White 2011). Specifically, lifetime users of steroids were about 4 times as likely to have used tobacco in the previous year; 6 times more likely to have used cannabis in the previous year; and 30 times more likely to have used cocaine or heroin (Dunn and White 2011). In a more recent study, males with high concerns about muscularity who used potentially unhealthy products to achieve their desired physiques were more likely than their peers to start binge drinking frequently. In addition, males with high concerns about muscularity and thinness, and those with high concerns about muscularity who used products to improve muscle size or strength were much more likely than their peers to start using drugs (Field et al. 2014).

A range of other high-risk behaviours have also been found to be high among adolescent steroid users. These include using injectable drugs, sharing needles, driving too fast, driving after drinking, carrying a gun, number of sexual partners in the past three months, injury sustained in a physical fight requiring medical attention, not wearing a helmet on motorcycle, and not wearing a seatbelt (Bahrke et al. 2000). Given that adolescence is a time of increased experimentation and risk taking, adolescents with high levels of body image concerns, may be especially vulnerable to health-risk behaviours. APEDs may also be used in the same way alcohol and other substances are used to cope with negative affect and low self-esteem (Ricciardelli and Williams 2011). In addition, some APEDs such as stimulants may be specifically used to suppress appetite and increase weight loss behaviours, in the way that smoking is used as a weight loss strategy (Warren et al. 2013).

More research is now needed to evaluate how APEDs may be used as mood-altering appetitive substances and the potential risk for adolescents' health and well-being (e.g. Hüsler and Plancherel 2006). More is known about alcohol as this is a commonly used/abused substance, and alcohol is generally accepted as a means of achieving 'felt' advantages with regard to mood repair, and is used as a means of temporary hedonic control over negative affect in general (Martens et al. 2008; Mason et al. 2008; Shaol et al. 2008). Outcome expectancies for alcohol use are often described as involving the enhancement of some aspect of self-presentation (e.g. social assertion, sexual functioning, tension reduction; Del Boca et al. 2002; Jones 2004; Morawska and Oei 2005), and thus it impacts on one's overall self-image, and more specifically, one's body image. Comparable outcomes expectancies for APEDs have yet to be investigated but we know that APEDs are used for promoting adolescents' self-image and body image. Clearly, this is an area where more research is also needed.

Negative affect and self-esteem. Closely related and often inter-related with body image concerns, substance abuse, and other risk-taking behaviours are negative affect and self-esteem. Negative affect encompasses mood states such as depression, anxiety, stress, shame, inadequacy, guilt and helplessness, and is closely associated with self-esteem and other self-concepts (Ricciardelli and McCabe 2001). Body-change strategies which result from body image concerns are often viewed as regulating and/or alleviating negative affect (Ricciardelli and McCabe 2004). Given that APEDs are also body-change strategies, their use may be viewed as a way of regulating and/or alleviating negative affect. Higher levels of depressive symptoms and lower self-esteem have been found to separate adolescent boys who use either steroids and/or food supplements versus those who do not (Smolak et al. 2005). Similarly, in a more recent study, feelings of sadness and hopelessness predicted both steroid and methamphetamine use among adolescent boys; and steroid use also predicted adolescents' consideration of suicide (Thorlton et al. 2012).

Other factors. The nature of the relationship that adolescents have with their parents is another factor that has been found to predict the use of food supplements (Ricciardelli and McCabe 2003). Ricciardelli and McCabe found that poor perceived parental relationship predicted adolescent boys' use of food supplements (e.g. protein powders) to change body weight among adolescent boys over an eight-month period (Ricciardelli and McCabe 2003). This measure of parent–adolescent relationships assessed how well adolescents thought they got along with their parents and the extent to which adolescents experienced parental acceptance and approval. Adolescents' relationships with opposite-gender peers are also important. As with parent relations, a more negative relationship with peers of the opposite gender has been found to predict the use of food supplements over an eight-month period (Ricciardelli and McCabe 2009). These findings are consistent with those reported in the review by Sagoe et al. (2014), which highlight that being more successful with the opposite gender is another important motivation for the initiation of steroid use.

The sporting environment, substance use, and other risk-taking behaviours, which are all associated with the use of APEDS, also reflect masculine gender-role stereotypes, norms and behaviours that are viewed as highly desirable for males (Ricciardelli and Williams 2011). Gender-role stereotypes more broadly reflect beliefs and behaviours typically attributed to men and women, which are learnt from an early age, and they have been shown to predict a range of health-risk behaviours including substance abuse and binge eating (Ricciardelli and Williams 2011). Gender-role stereotypes have yet to be specifically studied in relation to APEDs but their inclusion in future research will provide a sociocultural context for better understanding the reasons why many boys and adolescent males resort to APEDs.

Conclusions

In this chapter, we have reviewed the range of APEDs that boys and adolescent males use to improve their body image and appearance. These include steroids, steroid precursors such as creatine, but also stimulants, weight-loss supplements, and the abuse of prescription drugs for the purpose of weight loss. In addition, we have reviewed the range of risk factors associated with the use of APEDs. These, on the whole, are similar to the risk factors which have been found to be associated with disordered eating and other body-change strategies. Lastly, we have highlighted several areas where the findings are inconsistent and/or where further research is needed.

References

Almeida, S., Severo, M., Araújo, J., Lopes, C., & Ramos, E. (2012). Body image and depressive symptoms in 13-year-old adolescents. *Journal of Paediatrics and Child Health, 48*(10), E165–E171.

Bahrke, M. S., Yesalis, C. E., Kopstein, A. N., & Stephens, J. A. (2000). Risk factors associated with anabolic-androgenic steroid use among adolescents. *Sports Medicine, 29*(6), 397–405.

Coleman, J. (2011). *The nature of adolescence* (4th ed.). London: Routledge.
Del Boca, F. K., Darkes, J., Goldman, M. S., & Smith, G. (2002). Advancing the expectancy concept via the interplay between theory and research. *Alcoholism-Clinical and Experimental Research, 26*(6), 926–935.
Dunn, J., Lewis, V., & Patrick, S. (2010). The idealization of thin figures and appearance concerns in middle school children. *Journal of Applied Biobehavioral Research, 15*(3), 134–143.
Dunn, M., & White, V. (2011). The epidemiology of anabolic-androgenic steroid use among Australian secondary school students. *Journal of Science and Medicine in Sport, 14*(1), 10–14.
Eisenberg, M. E., Wall, M., & Neumark-Sztainer, D. (2012). Muscle-enhancing behaviors among adolescent girls and boys. *Pediatrics, 130*(6), 1019–1026.
Field, A. E., Austin, B., Carmargo, C. A., Barr Taylor, C., Striegel-Moore, R. H., Loud, K. J., et al. (2005). Exposure to the mass media, body shape concerns, and use of supplements to improve weight and shape among male and female adolescents. *Pediatrics, 116*(2), e214–e220.
Field, A. E., Camargo, C. A., Taylor, C. B., Berkey, C. S., Frazier, A. L., Gillman, M. W., et al. (1999). Overweight, weight concerns, and bulimic behaviors among girls and boys. *Journal of the Academy of Child and Adolescent Psychiatry, 38*(6), 754–760.
Field, A. E., Sonneville, K. R., Crosby, R. D., Swanson, S. A., Eddy, K. T., Camargo, C. A., et al. (2014). Prospective associations of concerns about physique and the development of obesity, binge drinking, and drug use among adolescent boys and young men. *JAMA Pediatrics, 168*(1), 34–39.
Grogan, S., & Richards, H. (2002). Body image: Focus groups with boys and men. *Men and Masculinities, 4*(3), 219–232.
Harmer, P. A. (2010). Anabolic-androgenic steroid use among young male and female athletes: Is the game to blame? *British Journal of Sports Medicine, 44*(1), 26–31.
Harrison, K., & Bond, B. J. (2007). Gaming magazines and the drive for muscularity in preadolescent boys: A longitudinal examination. *Body Image, 4*(3), 269–277.
Hildebrandt, T., Harty, S., & Langenbucher, J. W. (2012). Fitness supplements as a gateway for anabolic-androgenic steroid use. *Psychology of Addictive Behaviors, 26*(4), 955–962.
Holland, A., & Andre, T. (1994). Athletic participation and the social status of adolescent males and females. *Youth and Society, 25*(3), 388–407.

Huenemann, R. L., Shapiro, L. R., Hampton, M. D., & Mitchell, B. W. (1966). A longitudinal study of gross body composition and body conformation and association with food and activity in teenage population: Views of teenage subjects on body conformation, food and activity. *American Journal of Clinical Nutrition, 18*(5), 323–338.

Hüsler, G., & Plancherel, B. (2006). A gender specific model of substance abuse. *Addiction Research and Theory, 14*(4), 399–412.

Irving, L. M., Wall, M., Neumark-Sztainer, D., & Story, M. (2002). Steroid use among adolescents: Findings from Project EAT. *Journal of Adolescent Health, 30*(4), 243–252.

Jeffers, A. J., & Benotsch, E. G. (2014). Non-medical use of prescription stimulants for weight loss, disordered eating, and body image. *Eating Behaviors, 15*(3), 414–418.

Jeffers, A. J., Vataloro Hill, K. E., & Benotsch, E. G. (2014). Energy drinks, weight loss, and disordered eating behaviors. *Journal of American College Health, 62*(5), 336–342.

Jones, B. Y. (2004). Changing alcohol expectancies: techniques for altering motivations for drinking. In W. M. Cox & E. Klinger (Eds.), *Handbook of motivational counselling: Concepts, approaches and assessment* (pp. 373–387). Chichester: John Wiley.

Kanayama, G., Hudson, J. I., & Pope, H. G. (2012). Culture: Psychosomatics and substance abuse: The example of body image drugs. *Psychotherapy and Psychosomatics, 81*(2), 73–78.

Krowchuck, D. P., Kreiter, S. R., Woods, C. R., Sinal, S. H., & DuRant, R. H. (1998). Problem dieting behaviors among young adolescents. *Archives of Pediatrics and Adolescent Medicine, 152*(9), 884–889.

Labre, M. P. (2005). Burn fat, build muscle: A content analysis of men's heath and men's fitness. *International Journal of Men's Health, 4*(2), 187–200.

Lawler, M., & Nixon, E. (2011). Body dissatisfaction among adolescent boys and girls: The effects of body mass, peer appearance culture and internalization of appearance ideals. *Journal of Youth and Adolescence, 40*(1), 59–71.

Leit, R. A., Pope, H. G., & Gray, J. J. (2001). Cultural expectations of muscularity in the evolution of playgirl centerfolds. *International Journal of Eating Disorders, 29*(1), 90–93.

Lerner, R. M. (1972). "Richness" analyses of body build stereotype development. *Developmental Psychology, 7*(2), 219.

López-Guimeró, G., Neumark-Sztainer, D., Hannan, P., Fauquet, J., Loth, K., & Sánchz-Carracedo, D. (2013). Unhealthy weight-control behaviours, dieting and weight status: A cross-cultural comparison between North American and Spanish adolescents. *European Eating Disorders Review, 21*(4), 276–283.

Martens, M. P., Neighbors, C., Lewis, M. A., Lee, C. M., Oster-Aaland, L., & Larimer, M. E. (2008). The roles of negative affect and coping motives in the relationship between alcohol use and alcohol-related problems among college students. *Journal of Studies of Alcohol and Drugs, 69*(3), 412–419.

Martins, N., Williams, D. C., Ratan, R. A., & Harrison, K. (2010). Virtual muscularity: A content analysis of male video game characters. *Body Image, 8*(1), 43–51.

Mason, W. A., Hitchings, J. E., & Spoth, R. L. (2008). The interaction of conduct problems and depressed mood in relation to adolescent substance involvement and peer substance use. *Drug and Alcohol Dependence, 96*(3), 233–248.

McCabe, M. P., & Ricciardelli, L. A. (2004a). Body image dissatisfaction among males across the lifespan: A review of past literature. *Journal of Psychosomatic Research, 56*(6), 675–685.

McCabe, M. P., & Ricciardelli, L. A. (2004b). A longitudinal study of pubertal timing and extreme body change behaviors among adolescent boys and girls. *Adolescence, 39*(153), 145–166.

McCreary, D. R., & Sasse, D. K. (2000). An exploration of the drive for muscularity in adolescent boys and girls. *Journal of American College Health, 48*(6), 297–304.

Morawska, A., & Oei, T. P. S. (2005). Binge drinking in university students: A test of a cognitive model. *Addictive Behaviors, 30*(2), 203–218.

Morrison, T. G., & Halton, M. (2009). Buff, tough, and rough: Representations of muscularity in action motion pictures. *The Journal of Men' Studies, 17*(1), 57–74.

Neumark-Sztainer, D., Story, M., Falkner, N. H., Beuhring, T., & Resnick, M. D. (1999). Sociodemographic and personal characteristics of adolescents engaged in weight loss and weight/muscle gain behaviors: Who is doing what? *Preventative Medicine, 28*(1), 40–50.

Pope, H. G., Kanayama, G., & Hudson, J. I. (2012). Risk factors for illicit anabolic-androgenic steroid use in male weightlifters: A cross-sectional cohort study. *Biological Psychiatry, 71*(3), 254–261.

Pope, H. G., Olivardia, R., Gruber, A. J., & Borowiecki, J. J. (1999). Evolving ideals of male body image as seem through action toys. *International Journal of Eating Disorders, 26*(1), 65–72.

Ricciardelli, L. A., & McCabe, M. P. (2001). Self-esteem and negative affect as moderators of sociocultural influences on body dissatisfaction, strategies to decrease weight, and strategies to increase muscles among adolescent boys and girls. *Sex Roles, 44*(3–4), 189–207.

Ricciardelli, L. A., & McCabe, M. P. (2003). A longitudinal analysis of the role of biopsychosocial factors in predicting body change strategies among adolescent boys. *Sex Roles, 48*(7–8), 349–359.

Ricciardelli, L. A., & McCabe, M. P. (2004). A biopsychosocial model of disordered eating and the pursuit of muscularity in adolescent boys. *Psychological Bulletin, 130*(2), 179–205.

Ricciardelli, L. A., & McCabe, M. P. (2009). *Study of adolescent health risk behaviours*. Unpublished manuscript, Deakin University, Melbourne.

Ricciardelli, L. A., McCabe, M. P., Holt, K. E., & Finemore, J. (2003). A biopsychosocial model for understanding body image and body change strategies among children. *Journal of Applied Developmental Psychology, 24*(4), 475–495.

Ricciardelli, L. A., McCabe, M. P., & Ridge, D. (2006). The construction of the adolescent male body through sport. *Journal of Health Psychology, 11*(4), 577–587.

Ricciardelli, L. A., McCabe, M. P., Williams, R. J., & Thompson, J. K. (2007). The role of ethnicity and culture in body image and disordered eating among males. *Clinical Psychology Review, 27*(5), 582–606.

Ricciardelli, L. A., & Williams, R. J. (2011). The role of masculinity and femininity in the development and maintenance of health risk behaviors. In C. Blazina & D. S. Shen-Miller (Eds.), *An international psychology of men: Theoretical advances, case studies, and clinical innovation* (pp. 57–98). New York: Routledge.

Rodgers, R. F., Ganchou, C., Franko, D. L., & Chabro, H. (2012). Drive for muscularity and disordered eating among French adolescent males: A sociocultural model. *Body Image, 9*(3), 318–323.

Ross, H. E., & Ivis, F. (1999). Binge eating and substance use among male and female adolescents. *International Journal of Eating Disorders, 26*(3), 245–260.

Sagoe, D., Andreassen, C. S., & Pallesen, S. (2014). The aetiology and trajectory of anabolic-androgenic steroid used initiation: A systematic review and synthesis of qualitative research. *Substance Abuse Treatment, Prevention, and Policy, 9*(5), 283–396.

Shaol, G. D., Gudonis, L. C., Giancola, P. R., & Tarter, R. (2008). Negative affectivity and drinking in adolescents: An examination of moderators predicted by affect regulation theory. *Journal of Psychopathology and Behavioral Assessment, 30*(1), 61–70.

Smolak, L., Murnen, S. K., & Thompson, J. K. (2005). Sociocultural influences and muscle building in adolescent boys. *Psychology of Men and Masculinity, 6*(4), 227–239.

Stephen, E. M., Rose, J. S., Kenney, L., Rosselli-Navarra, F., & Weissman, R. S. Striegel (2014). Prevalence and correlates of unhealthy weight control behaviors; Findings from the national longitudinal study of adolescent health. *Journal of Eating Disorders, 2*. Viewed July 4, 2015, from http://www.jeatdisord.com/content/pdf/2050-2974-2-16.pdf

Tatangelo, G., & Ricciardelli, L. A. (2013). A qualitative study of preadolescent boys' and girls' body image: Gendered ideals and sociocultural influences. *Body Image, 10*(4), 591–598.

Thorlton, J. R., McElmurry, B., Park, C., & Hughes, T. (2012). Adolescent performance enhancing substance use: Regional differences across the US. *Journal of Addiction Nursing, 23*(2), 97–111.

van den Berg, P., Neumark-Sztainer, D., Cafri, G., & Wall, M. (2007). Steroid use among adolescents: Longitudinal findings from Project EAT. *Pediatrics, 119*(3), 476–486.

Vander Wal, J. S. (2011). Unhealthy weight control behaviors among adolescents. *Journal of Health Psychology, 17*(1), 110–120.

Warren, C. S., Lindsay, A. R., White, E. R., Claudat, K., & Velasquez, M. P. H. (2013). Weight-related concerns related to drug use for women in substance abuse treatment: Prevalence and relationships with eating pathology. *Journal of Substance Abuse Treatment, 44*(5), 494–501.

Whitaker, A., Davies, M., Shaffer, D., Johnson, J., Abramam, S., Walsh, B. T., et al. (1989). The struggle to be thin: A survey of anorexic and bulimic symptoms in a non-referred adolescent population. *Psychological Medicine, 19*(1), 143–163.

White, S. A., Duda, J. L., & Keller, M. R. (1998). The relationship between goal orientation and perceived purposes of sport among youth sport participants. *Journal of Sport Behavior, 21*(4), 475–483.

Yager, Z., & O'Dea, J. A. (2014). Relationships between body image, nutritional supplement us, and attitudes towards doping in sport among adolescents boys: Implications for prevention programs. *Journal of the International Society for Sports Nutrition, 11*. Viewed June 23, 2015, from http://link.springer.com/article/10.1186/1550-2783-11-13#page-1

3

Muscle Dysmorphia and Anabolic-Androgenic Steroid Use

Dave Smith, Mary Caitlyn Rutty, and Tracy W. Olrich

Background

Historically, public health guidelines promote the addition of physical activity exemplified in terms of aerobic exercise and resistance training for cardiorespiratory fitness and musculoskeletal health. The exercise prescription is seen as an aid in preventive disease medicine (Winett and Carpinelli 2001), an activity to increase self-esteem (Spence et al. 2005), and is used in a variety of psychiatric therapeutic interventions. However, when exercise is performed excessively, the practice can adapt as a pathological association of body image disorders. This association has

D. Smith (✉)
MMU Cheshire, Exercise and Sport Science, Crewe Green Road, CW1 5DU Crewe, Cheshire, UK

M.C. Rutty
Mill, 31241, 48066 Roseville, MI, USA

T.W. Olrich
Physical Education and Sport, Central Michigan University, 131 Foust Hall, 48859 Mt. Pleasant, MI, USA

© The Editor(s) (if applicable) and The Author(s) 2016
M. Hall et al. (eds.), *Chemically Modified Bodies*,
DOI 10.1057/978-1-137-53535-1_3

been confined traditionally to the relationship between aerobic exercise and eating disorders in women who aspire an unattainable thin physique (Murray and Baghurst 2013). Research has currently illustrated a growing prevalence of body image dissatisfaction among men, which posits that both males as young as 6 years reportedly desire a physique that differs from their current perceptions of self (Pope et al. 2000). College aged men reported that the ideal masculine body carries, on average, 25 pounds more muscle than their own physique (Olivardia et al. 2004). In addition, males as a cohort desire to gain approximately 17 pounds of muscle mass, regardless of their current shape (Pope et al. 2000).

The reasons for this apparently increasing trend towards increasing body dissatisfaction amongst males may lie in the increasing promotion of lean, heavily muscled body as the male ideal (Grieve 2007). Mesomorphic males are viewed as more socially desirable and possessing greater physical and athletic prowess than ectomorphic males (Pope et al. 2000). At the same time, over recent decades the cultural norm for the ideal male physique has become increasingly more muscular (Leit et al. 2001). Therefore, it is perhaps not surprising that an increasing number of males report body dissatisfaction (Phillips and Drummond 2001) and an increased desire for a lean, heavily muscled physique (Leone et al. 2005). A recent survey (Field et al. 2014) found that almost 18 % of adolescent boys were concerned about not being muscular enough; perhaps not surprising when even toy action figures have increased in muscularity in recent years to the point where they have physiques that in many cases would be unattainable even for the most advanced bodybuilders (Baghurst et al. 2006).

Given the aforementioned argument, we argue that body image dissatisfaction should be a concern to all those interested in mental health. The following sections of this chapter describe how such dissatisfaction drives physique-enhancing behaviours that can reach clinical and debilitating levels. Firstly, relevant psychiatric disorders of body dysmorphic disorder and MD will be explained, and the relationship between MD and the use of physique-enhancing drugs will be explored. Psychological and sociocultural factors influencing this relationship will be examined, and suggestions made for future research.

Body Dysmorphic Disorder and Muscle Dysmorphia

BDD is a severe psychiatric disorder characterized by time-consuming preoccupations with one or more perceived defects or flaws in appearance that are not observable or appear slight to others (Kelly et al. 2014). BDD-related preoccupations cause clinically significant distress or impairment in functioning. BDD is often accompanied by repetitive behaviours or mental acts that occur in response to the appearance preoccupations (e.g. mirror checking, skin picking, excessive grooming, comparing with others; American Psychiatric Association 2013; Phillips et al. 2005). Muscle dysmorphia (MD) represents the pathological pursuit of muscularity and is characterized by an intensely distressing preoccupation that one is of insufficient muscularity (although appearing normal or muscular) coupled with rigorous exercise and dietary practices that take precedence over other important areas of life. As a subtype of BDD, MD is unique in its form of causing preoccupation with the body as a whole, instead of a specific body part as seen in typical BDD.

MD was first noted in research as 'reverse anorexia' (Pope et al. 1993) and explained as the male version of the disorder anorexia nervosa, much like the female's need for thinness, as males experiencing this disorder are often concerned with losing weight (Murray et al. 2010). However, it was also recognized that minimizing body fat and maximizing muscularity is the generalized need or want by those with MD, rather than solely the fear of losing mass. As noted in our introduction, pressure has increased for the male ideal body type to appear muscular, inversely related to the ideal female body type (appearing thin). This pressure has aided in men and women feeling dissatisfied in the way their bodies appear, and in some cases a distorted body image is experienced. As a result, affected individuals may neglect important social or occupational activities because of shame over their perceived appearance flaws or their need to attend to a meticulous diet and time-consuming workout schedule (Pope et al. 2005).

Diagnostic Criteria

A coherent line of research emerged after the introduction of the concept of reverse anorexia, and the term 'muscle dysmorphia' was first introduced by Pope Jr. et al. (1997), along with a series of diagnostic criteria for the disorder. The concept of MD was proposed as a form of BDD as it was found in Pope et al.'s study that 9.3 % of 193 individuals with already diagnosed BDD portrayed associated features of what would be explained as MD. The essential feature of MD is characterized as the severe need to be overly muscular and lean, which in turn causes significant impairment and distress in daily life. The symptoms of the disorder cause a distortion of reality and individuals with MD obsessively compare themselves to others with the notion that in most cases, they are inadequately small, despite realistic existence. It is frequently observed that individuals with MD will feel levels of extreme embarrassment and anxiety when forced to present their body in the public eye.

Following the early research, MD was recognized in the *Diagnostic and Statistical Manual of Mental Disorders: Text Revision* (American Psychiatric Association 2000; DSM-IV) as a subtype of BDD categorized in the somatoform spectrum, a type of mental illness that causes physical bodily symptoms. As research continued, no evidence for MD relating to a somatoform disorder was found, and in the DSM-V, published in 2013, the diagnosis of MD now lies in the obsessive-compulsive spectrum as a subtype of BDD.

Cafri et al. (2008) and Olivardia et al. (2000) revealed that symptoms of MD start manifesting at about 19.5 years of age. The symptoms of MD these authors noted were as follows: compulsive mirror checking, extensive time spent exercising, thinking about their muscularity >30 times a day, avoidance of people, places, and activities related to their body appearance, and abuse of performance-enhancing drugs. Additionally, Cafri et al. (2008) found that 67 % of their subjects with MD reportedly thought about their muscularity more than 3 hours daily. It is well documented that MD affects an individual on a behavioural, cognitive, and social level. Behavioural symptoms studied include pharmacological use, workout rituals, supplement use, and dietary behaviour. Psychological factors include exercise dependence, and protection of physique and body size/symmetry (Rohman 2009). When MD behaviour characteristics continue to grow in an individual, negative consequences such as alienation, narcissism, and positive deviance may develop.

Another diagnostic specific of MD is the presence of comorbid psychological disorders. MD has been associated with higher rates of lifetime mood disorders such as major depressive disorder (Wolke and Sapouna 2008). Anxiety disorders have also been associated with the development of MD such as panic disorder, posttraumatic stress disorder, obsessive-compulsive disorder (OCD), and generalized anxiety disorder (Cafri et al. 2008). In fact, MD has also been categorized as a subtype of OCD. OCD as a form of anxiety encompasses obsessive rituals to overcome levels of anxious distress. The compulsive rituals in MD include the overwhelming time spent training in exercise, nutrition, and the use of performance-enhancing drugs to aid in muscular development; it is the ritualistic nature of behaviours performed to alleviate levels of physique-related anxiety in MD that has led to such an association.

Approaches began comparing MD and the pathology following that of an eating disorder, and the most recent literature revisits the association. Researchers have proposed that MD presentations of body dysmorphic disorder do not generally include food and exercise-related psychopathology, and the diagnostic criteria for body dysmorphic disorder posit that those experiencing such concerns, in conjunction with shape-related body image and weight distortion, are best accounted for by an eating disorder diagnosis (Murray and Touyz 2013). Scopes have, therefore, reanalyzed MD through the lens of an eating disorder and found that levels of functional impairment have closely aligned.

Perhaps the most comprehensive attempt to date to provide an all-encompassing model of MD has been that of Lantz et al. (2001), whose conceptual model included many of the factors noted earlier. They identified two precipitating factors, *self-esteem* and *body dissatisfaction*, that increase motivation to engage in exercise aimed at physique development. The development of muscle then increases self-esteem, which will increase commitment to the exercise regime. This is problematic if a person's self-esteem becomes dependent on this connection.

The six behavioural characteristics that develop from MD, according to Lantz et al.'s model, include *body size/symmetry* (e.g. concern with developing an 'ideal' muscular body), *dietary constraints* (e.g. consumption of an optimal 'muscle building' diet), *physique protection* (e.g. hiding the physique with baggy clothing), *supplement use* (e.g. protein supplements), *pharmacological abuse* (e.g. use of anabolic-androgenic steroids), and *exercise dependence* (i.e. compulsive exercise). Each characteristic could then maintain a cyclical influence of more pathological behaviours. For example, as a person's attitude towards his or her body becomes more pathological, he or she may begin to experiment with muscle-building drugs. As his or her physique develops, he or she will associate this with the pharmacological intervention, and so that behaviour is increasingly reinforced.

The overall prevalence of MD is under researched yet estimated by Olivardia (2007) as 100,000 cases in the USA. It was noted that there is an assumption that a much larger quantity of individuals experience less severe versions of the disorder. Females have been found to experience most forms of BDD, yet MD has been found to be more prevalent in men. The natures of MD and BDD are such that individuals will likely not admit their disorder, or seek help, because of embarrassment. This makes it difficult to accurately estimate a prevalence of BDD and MD.

Muscle Dysmorphia and Bodybuilding/Weightlifting

It is important to note the difference between 'bodybuilders' and 'weight lifters', as both terms are often used interchangeably. A weight lifter is an individual who undergoes the process of exercise in the form of resistance training to control and develop strength (and sometimes musculature), but where lifting heavy weights is considered an end in itself. In contrast, although bodybuilders also lift weights, the end purpose of this is purely to develop their musculature. Also, competitive bodybuilders participate in competitions where they display their physiques. Bodybuilders have been found to carry the highest level of body dissatisfaction compared to other competitive athletic groups (Blouin and Goldfield 1995), and are the main group examined in MD literature.

Most of those susceptible to MD start lifting weights in their adolescent years in the hope of building a muscular physique to cover up their inner insecurities. However, even after attaining considerable muscle mass, the insecurities persist (Rohman 2009). The research question naturally arises whether participation in lifting weights and/or bodybuilding is a precursor to developing body image pathology and increasingly into BDD/MD? This was addressed in Olivardia et al.'s (2000) study when comparing 24 men with MD and 30 normal weight lifters. The men with MD differed significantly on measures of body dissatisfaction, eating behaviours, prevalence of steroid usage, and lifetime prevalence of DSV-IV related mood, anxiety, and eating disorders. It was found that the normal weight lifters portrayed little psychopathology compared to the weight lifters with MD.

Individuals with MD are distinct from normal weight lifters in their symptom pathology and psychiatric comorbidity (Cafri et al. 2008). For weight lifters to be diagnosed with MD, they must show a level of functional impairment. Those with the disorder have reported lifting weights 7 days a week and more than once a day for an hour and a half at each session, which is a much higher amount of training than in a typical weightlifting routine. They tend to deny occupational opportunities because holding a job does not allow them to engage in extensive weight lifting and eating habits, which are a priority in the functioning of their lives (e.g. see Fussell 1991). Others have explained that living alone also diminishes stress of a significant other tampering with their strict regime. Therefore, there should not be confusion between mere enthusiasm and a strictly dedicated lifestyle of bodybuilding and MD. The difference lies in profound levels of extreme distress and maladaptive coping behaviours.

Muscle Dysmorphia and Performance-Enhancing Drugs

Referring to the first published study on MD (or 'reverse anorexia' as it was referred to by Pope et al. 1993), all nine participants then who were found to portray to what would later be developed as MD were using anabolic-androgenic steroids (AAS). Research began exploring this association and amongst the many rituals to require more mass found in those with MD, the use of AAS has been the most frequently associated. Many report that use of AAS is aimed at curing their disorder, yet others have explained that the use of the steroids aided in the development of their hyper-mesomorphic physique preoccupation.

To appreciate the role that AAS may play in the lives of those experiencing MD, an understanding of the impact AAS use has on those choosing to use is needed. Sagoe et al. (2014) conducted a literature review of 44 qualitative studies concerning AAS use, and found a myriad of reasons for initiating use. However, the three main reasons for initiation of use were: (1) wanting success in sports participation (particularly power sports), (2) to overcome negative body image, and (3) dealing with psychological disorders such as depression.

Once AAS use was initiated, several studies (Olrich 1993; Olrich and Ewing 1999; Petrocelli et al. 2008; Vassallo and Olrich 2010) found the AAS use period to have a profound impact on the users. Users experienced significant positive increases in muscle mass, strength, and self-confidence, which will be discussed later in the text and will draw heavily from research conducted by the authors of this chapter.

Perceived benefits of AAS use. In a study of competitive and non-competitive bodybuilders, Olrich and Ewing (1999) reported that 9 of 10 AAS users spoke of the AAS use period in very positive terms, while in a study of former collegiate athletes, Vassallo and Olrich (2010) found all 38 participants perceived their AAS use period positively. Participants using AAS experienced rapid and profound increases in strength, power, and muscle mass. Those gains led to a number of positive corollary benefits, including greater peer recognition, greater perceived sexual attractiveness, and greater success in sport. The following responses capture such positive benefits:

> Physically, stronger. I felt like training all the time. I loved coming into the gym, because I could hoist all these heavy poundages. I was making good gains. The pump I got was incredible. When you get pumped, I mean you could see man, you're looking huge and ripped. And it was just unbelievable. It really motivated you to get into the gym (Olrich 1993).
>
> I am personally a lot more energetic and aggressive, probably a combination of those two words. Needless to say, I'm a lot more confident and potentially cocky for the fact that what happens is I'm looking physically better, be it bloated or not. I tend to be a bit more cut when I'm on drugs, so I tend to look a little better. My muscular definition is coming out, my strength is increasing, so each time (I'm in the gym) I try to obtain a new goal. I'm obtaining goals and as with anyone in life, when you try for something to obtain goals, you feel great. You feel great because you can do it. I can do anything. I'm more horny. I'm more aggressive. I just tend to attack things a lot more and everything seems to be clicking. I feel better. I'm stronger. You do, you have to sleep because you're training hard, but you don't feel like you have to have as much sleep. You tend to be on top of the world. I don't know, I guess I like that feeling (Olrich and Ewing 1999).
>
> Oh, positive for sure. Because I kept my spot in baseball, and I developed a chiseled body, and my grades went through the roof. I never got a better grade point than during those semesters I used the juice (Vassallo and Olrich 2010).

As these quotes point out, the AAS use experience had a powerful effect on these men, and the benefits went well beyond the walls of the gym. Further, the men perceived significant increases in self-confidence and peer recognition. The following quotes were from athletes who used during their college sporting career as reported by Vassallo and Olrich (2010) when asked if their levels of confidence were impacted by AAS use:

> Is the Pope catholic? Of course they were. That was the sole reason I took three more cycles throughout college. I felt like I was on top of the world anytime I was on the juice.

Another of the participants had this to say:

> (Levels of confidence) They were as big as the frickin sky. I was the man and you better bring your best or I would rip your f—g head off. I knew that when I was on the 'roids I could do some major hitting compared to when I was off the shit. I, you know, I was meaner than hell and I needed those things to help me get that edge.

And another stated:

> I was, I don't know if this is proper, but I felt like the f—g man. I mean I was just invincible. I felt I could do anything I put my mind to, and 9 times out of 10 I did. That was the best I ever felt about myself. Man, I miss that feeling.

And the statement by another participant captured the sentiment well:

> That is an understatement if I ever heard one before. I mean I felt like I could climb the tallest mountain with no training if I needed to. I know that is a stupid analogy. But I was more confident than I ever was in my life when I was on the steroids. I am a very confident individual without the 'roids (sic) and when I was on the stuff it was absolutely amazing how my confidence levels just soared through the roof. I loved that feeling.

Similar responses were found with competitive and recreational bodybuilders (Olrich and Ewing 1999):

> Oh yeah. King of the world, it's just a good feeling. You can just think straight. It's just a good feeling. But you just feel ... you just think differently about situations. You react differently. You feel good about yourself, and you know you've got the edge. And that affects you through your whole cycle, whether you're training or not. You've got the edge.

Perceived positive increases in both self-image and self-confidence were also due to peer recognition which many of the participants discussed.

3 Muscle Dysmorphia and Anabolic-Androgenic Steroid Use

When you're on steroids, if you're bigger, you're stronger, and you're getting personal recognition from your peers ... you're enjoying it. You're enjoying the peer recognition. If you're on steroids, and because you're on steroids you grow, people are noticing you. You're lifting more weight, or whatever the scenario is, that you're getting more peer recognition.

AAS and Psychological Addiction. Participants in these studies (Olrich 1993; Olrich and Ewing 1999; Olrich and Vassallo 2006; Vassallo and Olrich 2010) were queried concerning their perceptions as to whether AAS had any potential to be psychologically addictive. Not surprisingly, considering the aforementioned responses, all of the men interviewed believed that AAS had a strong potential for psychological addiction, whether the men believed they experienced such an addiction or not. Representative statements from the bodybuilders are given next:

Sure. I know definitely there is (a psychological dependence). There's definitely. I know that. I know for a fact that, because I have troubles when I do a cycle coming off. Because you see, you like how they make you feel, okay? Mentally, they just do something to you. You feel great. And then you get so much stronger. And you blow right up. And you puff up, you know. And you look good. And you put on the weight. And that's what bodybuilders wants to do the most, is that you get that weight. And you want to get that weight up. And it comes like nothing man. And it's just there. And then it goes. Just like it came. You keep some, but you lose the majority. You do keep some. And you lose the edge. You lose that strength, that cockiness. You know, all the good things that come, that you feel from them, just go away.

Another bodybuilder spoke in a similar manner, but discussed the role of peer recognition in the process:

I've never been on drugs where, "Oh my God, I have to have a shot, or I have to have a pill." I've never met anybody that's that way. But, they definitely want the effects of being big, because of the side effects of that. The side effects being that they are getting peer recognition or personal recognition of some sort. "God, you're really growing," "God, you look great."

"God, you're stronger than shit." People thrive off that, and you can't tell me in our society that people don't thrive off of recognition.

The former collegiate athletes of Vassallo and Olrich (2010) also spoke to the strength of this perceived, powerful dependency to AAS. One of the former football players stated:

> Of course there is man (a psychological addiction). I mean that is the main reason that me and my friends would do the shit again and again. We missed the feeling it gives you against your opponent. It was f—g awesome. Yeah, the strength you get is great, but the reason I did the shit time and again was due to the fact that I wanted the mental edge it gives you.

Another football player who had also experimented with a variety of recreational drugs stated how he felt the addictive qualities of AAS were stronger than any other substance he had tried (Olrich and Vassallo 2006).

> I know this sounds crazy, but I really think that they are more addictive than any recreational drug I have tried in my life. I mean once you have that feeling of invincibility you never want it to go away. It was something I needed more and more the older I got. I mean the last four cycles that I did (during his college career) was due to the fact that I missed the mental edge that I had over my opponent.

Another powerful statement from a former athlete is given next:

> There definitely is an addiction there that affects your mind. I think it is because the stuff gives you a mental edge that you will never experience in your life unless you do the stuff. I know it is not easy for someone to believe, but I promise you that the stuff gives you a mental boost in everything you do. It is f—ing awesome. I hope people realize that this is why the majority of people decide to do the stuff more and more. It just seems to give you an edge that is far more than the physical aspect that everyone thinks about. Physical strength you get from the stuff is great. But I promise you the stuff that you miss when you are done with your cycle is the edge that the stuff gives you in the head.

The AAS use experience and muscle dysmorphia. The participants quoted in the studies discussed earlier were not assessed for MD. Yet, the nature of comments given by the participants shows the profound impact AAS would likely have on those who may have such a condition. The men had seemingly profound increases in strength, power, muscle mass, self-confidence, and they felt mentally they had 'the edge'. As the men discussed, the impact of AAS was felt throughout all aspects of their lives. Their perceptions of psychological addiction to AAS were insightful, noting the breadth of the impact of AAS on their lives and how that contributed to the addictive nature of the substances. Given this, it is not surprising that as noted earlier studies have found that many of those exhibiting symptoms of MD are AAS users, and indeed Lantz et al.'s (2001) conceptual model of MD includes pharmacological use as one of the behaviours that characterizes those with MD. Cafri et al. (2005) also suggested that MD often culminates in AAS use to try to increase muscularity. The findings of Davies et al. (2011) seem to support the idea that steroids are often used for this purpose, and also suggest that they may be successful in this regard for some bodybuilders. In this study, interviews were conducted with current and former AAS users to explore symptoms of MD. Interestingly, the current users were generally happy with their physiques, whereas body dissatisfaction was much more evident in the former users and they were more likely to engage in physique protection behaviours. Also, symptoms of exercise dependence were more prevalent in the former users, which the authors attributed to the fact that they were no longer using AAS so felt they had to work harder to maintain their size. Indeed, two of the former users interviewed were considering re-using the drugs as they felt they looked better when taking them.

Thus, there is some evidence that the use of AAS may be motivated by feelings of MD, and also that AAS use is associated with improved body satisfaction, but that this evaporates with cessation of use as the muscular gains produced by the drugs diminish. Given that AAS users appear to mostly view the experience of AAS use as positive despite the attendant health risks, and that recidivism is common in former users, trying to persuade users that such use is not in their best interests may be very challenging. Also, treating those with symptoms of MD is complicated by the often attendant drug use. The following section will explore the treatment issue and offer some tentative suggestions.

Treatment of Those with Muscle Dysmorphia

There are a number of challenging barriers to overcome in treating MD. The first one of these is that the vast majority of individuals with MD will not seek treatment (Pope et al. 2000). It is traditionally seen as vain for males to be concerned about their body's appearance, and therefore, they may well be reluctant to open up to others about their body image concerns or even to admit them to themselves. They are likely to present to medical doctors for other reasons, such as weight training injuries, or concern regarding health issues relating to their AAS use. It is therefore important that GPs, physiotherapists, and other health professionals are made aware of the symptoms of MD so they can recognize it in their patients. Competitive bodybuilders with symptoms of MD may present to coaches or sport psychologists for performance enhancement issues, so again it is important that the coach and sport psychologist can identify and understand this issue. The crucial thing here is for such professionals to encourage individuals to talk openly about body image concerns and show understanding that such concerns are perfectly normal and indeed commonplace. Another factor that can make MD difficult to treat is the harmful and unrealistic portrayal of the human body in the media and society at large; the increasingly muscular portrayal of the male physique noted earlier not only makes MD more likely to occur, but also makes it difficult to treat. Given the pervasiveness of muscular images, from action toys to male models and even movie stars (including many AAS users), individuals are constantly reminded that their physiques do not seem to 'measure up', and thus messages from professionals who are trying to treat an individual with MD have to compete against these much more pervasive and alluring ones.

That said, it is far from the case that there is nothing that psychologists, psychiatrists, and other health professionals can do. Appropriate counseling may be very helpful here, for example. Body dissatisfaction can be tackled by helping to reshape the individual's distorted body image; if the individual can be encouraged to realize that media-presented images of the human body are not the norm and are indeed unattainable for the vast majority of people, this could be very helpful (Leone et al. 2005).

Given that MD is associated with low self-esteem (Wolke and Sapouna 2008), strategies to enhance self-esteem will likely also prove useful. It is important for such individuals to develop non-appearance based sources of self-esteem so they do not judge their worth as a human being solely through their muscularity. Developing other interests that can serve as sources of self-esteem may be crucial in weaning people off some of the unhealthy behaviours that occur with MD. Indeed, Vassallo and Olrich (2010) found that when AAS users developed other important life roles such as husband, father, and businessman, they ceased AAS use as having a muscular physique was not seen as important to them any more. It should be recognized that individuals presenting with MD symptoms may not be at the point where they have other life roles that could easily replace that of 'bodybuilder', but certainly appropriate counseling may help individuals get to this point. Given that MD is strongly correlated with concurrent anxiety (Wolke and Sapouna 2008), the psychologist should also teach coping strategies to ensure that MD-susceptible individuals are less likely to rely on maladaptive and unhealthy coping strategies such as AAS use.

It is important, however, that counseling is done in such a way that it is sympathetic to the individual's desire to achieve or maintain a high level of muscularity. Individuals with MD may worry that the healthcare professional may try to take away their ways of coping with their MD, such as extreme amounts of exercise, fad diets, and drug use. Thus, simple suggestions made to them that they should stop such practices, with nothing to replace them that would help them maintain their quest for a muscular physique, are likely to fall on deaf ears. So, for example, such individuals could be advised to consult a qualified sports nutritionist to help them develop a healthy muscle-building diet, and to possibly change their workout environment away from a 'hardcore' bodybuilding gym, which is an environment in which AAS use and obsessive and unhealthy training regimens often begin. As noted by Smith et al. (2009), the social environment in such gyms often encourages and reinforces the use of AAS, for example, and as such gyms typically contain AAS users, then this may also normalize the steroid-using physique to the other gym users. In addition, many AAS users purchase the drugs in these gyms (Smith et al. 2009). Therefore, other options should be examined such as facilities with a broader range of clientele, or home training.

Such strategies may help reduce the likelihood of AAS use, but care needs to be taken with those who are already using such drugs. Abrupt cessation of AAS use can lead to suicidal ideation (Thiblin et al. 1999), possibly due to testosterone levels becoming much lower than baseline, leading to depression. Therefore, when ceasing use AAS users should be referred to a physician with expertise in this area who can advise them on how best to cycle gradually off of AAS. Many bodybuilders use human chorionic gonadotrophin to maintain testosterone production when cycling off AAS use and thus avoid these problems; however, the effectiveness and safety of this still needs to be assessed in clinical research.

Interestingly, Pope et al. (2000) report some individuals with MD being successfully treated with antidepressants such as fluoxitine. Unfortunately, the use of these drugs has been shown to lead to suicidal ideation in some patients (e.g. Mann and Kapur 1991), and therefore, given that the lower testosterone levels may already lead to depression when cycling off AAS, the use of such antidepressants may prove especially dangerous. Therefore, prescribing such drugs when individuals are coming off AAS is likely unwise.

Conclusion

Individuals exhibiting symptoms of MD often use AAS and other substances to try to achieve or maintain a hyper-mesomorphic physique. The effects of these drugs can serve as a powerful reinforcer of this behaviour given these individuals' insecurities regarding their muscularity. Also, there is some evidence that individuals who do stop using AAS report increased symptoms of MD following cessation, due to the loss of muscle mass. Therefore, recidivism is likely high in this population, and simple messages that the use of such drugs can damage long-term health are unlikely on their own to be effective in this population. Particular care must be taken with those who have ceased AAS use to encourage them to develop other interests that may at least reduce their reliance on their body as their sole source of self-esteem. Given that the gym environment can normalize and reinforce both feelings of MD and AAS use, affected individuals should be encouraged to find a less 'hardcore' training environment where they will be exposed to a broader range of clientele. Advice from a qualified nutritionist on dieting to optimize lean muscle mass may also help here. Though some success has been found with the use of antidepressants, caution should be exercised with these as, especially combined with the low testosterone levels that result from cycling off of AAS, suicidal ideation can result in some individuals.

Since the early research of Pope et al., our understanding of MD and AAS use has been greatly improved. However, there are a number of issues that merit further exploration. Given that we now have 60 years' worth of current and former AAS users, large scale research with this fascinating (and large) group of people is possible. For example, it would be useful to explore the characteristics of MD with former AAS users to see if they self-identify particular times in their lives when they behaved in such ways and suffered from MD. This would help us to understand whether MD is associated with certain life stages, or if it is something individuals struggle with for a lifetime. The issue of other roles in the person's life becoming more important, and thus the person beginning to identify more strongly with later emerging roles and less strongly with that of 'bodybuilder' and 'steroid user', may be particularly important here. It is well worth exploring given its potential importance in developing strategies to combat MD and AAS use. We could also ask individuals identify strategies they may have used to combat MD, if in fact they had. This could become invaluable information for those attempting to counsel MD-affected/AAS-using individuals. Indeed, given the large amount of qualitative research published on this topic, it is very interesting that relatively little attention has been paid to how individuals have attempted to overcome feelings of MD; we think it is time for an exploration of this key issue.

References

American Psychiatric Association. (2013). *American Psychiatric Association Diagnostic and statistical manual of mental disorders* (5th ed.). Washington, DC: Author.

Baghurst, T., Hollander, D. B., Nardella, B., & Haff, G. (2006). Change in sociocultural ideal male physique: An examination of past and present action figures. *Body Image, 3,* 87–91.

Blouin, A., & Goldfield, G. (1995). Body image and steroid use in male bodybuilders. *International Journal of Eating Disorders, 18*, 159–165.

Cafri, G., Olivardia, R., & Thompson, J. (2008). Symptom characteristics and psychiatric comorbidity among males with muscle dysmorphia. *Comprehensive Psychiatry, 49*, 374–379.

Cafri, G., Thompson, J., Ricciardelli, L., McCabe, M., Smolak, L., & Yesalis, C. (2005). Pursuit of the muscular ideal: Physical and psychological consequences and putative risk factors. *Clinical Psychology Review, 25*, 215–239.

Davies, R., Smith, D., & Collier, K. (2011). Muscle dysmorphia among current and former steroid users. *Journal of Clinical Sport Psychology, 5*, 77–94.

Field, E., Sonneville, K., Crosby, R., Swanson, S., Eddy, K., Camargo, C., et al. (2014). Prospective associations of concerns about physique and the development of obesity, binge drinking and drug use among adolescent boys and young adult men. *Journal of the American Medical Association, 168*, 34–39.

Fussell, S. (1991). *Muscle: Confessions of an unlikely bodybuilder*. London: Abacus.

Grieve, F. G. (2007). A conceptual model of factors leading to the development of muscle dysmorphia. *Eating Disorders: The Journal of Treatment and Prevention, 15*, 63–80.

Kelly, M., Didie, E., & Phillips, K. (2014). Personal and appearance-based rejection sensitivity in body dysmorphic disorder. *Body Image, 11*, 260–265.

Lantz, C. D., Rhea, D. J., & Mayhew, J. L. (2001). *The drive for size: A psychobehavioral model of muscle dysmorphia* (pp. 71–86). Winter: International Sports Journal.

Leit, R. A., Gray, J. J., & Pope Jr., H. G. (2001). The media's representation of the ideal male body: A cause for muscle dysmorphia? *International Journal of Eating Disorders, 31*, 334–338.

Leone, J., Sedory, E., & Gray, K. (2005). Recognition and treatment of muscle dysmorphia and related body image disorders. *Journal of Athletic Training, 40*, 352–359.

Mann, J. J., & Kapur, S. (1991). The emergence of suicidal ideation and behaviour during antidepressant pharmacology. *Archives of General Psychiatry, 48*, 1027–1033.

Murray, S., & Baghurst, T. (2013). Revisiting the diagnostic criteria for muscle dysmorphia. *Strength and Conditioning Journal, 35*, 69–74.

Murray, S., Rieger, E., Touyz, S. W., & De La Garza Garcia, Y. (2010). Muscle dysmorphia and the DSM-V conundrum: Where does it belong? A review paper. *International Journal of Eating Disorders, 43*(6), 483–491.

Murray, S., & Touyz, S. W. (2013). Muscle dysmorphia: Towards a diagnostic consensus. *Australian and New Zealand Journal of Psychiatry, 47*, 206–207.
Olivardia, R. (2007). Muscle dysmorphia: Characteristics, assessment, and treatment. In *The muscular ideal: Psychological, social, and medical perspectives*. American Psychological Association, Washington, DC, 123–139.
Olivardia, R., Pope Jr., H. G., Borowiecki, J. J., & Cohane, G. H. (2004). Biceps and body image: The relationship between muscularity and self-esteem, depression, and eating disorder symptoms. *Psychology of Men & Masculinity, 5*, 112–120.
Olivardia, R., Pope Jr., H. G., & Hudson, J. I. (2000). Muscle dysmorphia in male weightlifters: A case-control study. *The American Journal of Psychiatry, 157*(8), 1291–1296.
Olrich, T. W. (1993). The relationship of male identity, the mesomorphic image, and anabolic steroid use in bodybuilding. *International Institute for Sport and Human Performance Microforms Publications, 7*, 1673.
Olrich, T. W., & Martha, E. E. (1999). Life on steroids: Bodybuilders describe their perceptions of the anabolic-androgenic steroid use period. *Sport Psychologist, 13*(3), 299–312.
Olrich, T. W., & Vassallo, M. (2006). Psychological addiction to anabolic steroids: Exploring the role of social mediation. *New England Law Review, 40*, 735–746.
Petrocelli, M., Oberweis, T., & Petrocelli, J. (2008). Getting huge, getting ripped: A qualitative exploration of recreational steroid use. *Journal of Drug Issues, 38*, 1187–1205.
Phillips, J. M., & Drummond, M. J. (2001). An investigation into body image perception, body satisfaction and exercise expectation of male fitness leaders: Implications for professional practice. *Leisure Studies, 20*, 95–105.
Phillips, K. A., Menard, W., Fay, C., & Pagano, M. E. (2005). Psychosocial functioning and quality of life in body dysmorphic disorder. *Comprehensive Psychiatry, 46*, 254–260.
Pope, C. G., Pope, H. G., Menard, W., Fay, C., Olivardia, R., & Phillips, K. A. (2005). Clinical features of muscle dysmorphia among males with body dysmorphic disorder. *Body Image, 2*, 395–400.
Pope Jr., H. G., Gruber, A. J., Choi, P., Olivardia, P. R., & Phillips, K. A. (1997). Muscle dysmorphia: An underrecognized form of body dysmorphic disorder. *Psychosomatics: Journal of Consultation and Liaison Psychiatry, 38*, 548–557.
Pope, H. G., Katz, D. L., & Hudson, J. I. (1993). Anorexia nervosa and "reverse anorexia" among 108 male bodybuilders. *Comprehensive Psychiatry, 34*, 406–409.

Pope, H. G., Phillips, K. A., & Olivardia, R. (2000). *The adonis complex: The secret crisis of male body image obsession*. New York: Free Press.

Rohman, L. (2009). The relationship between anabolic androgenic steroids and muscle dysmorphia: A review. *Eating Disorders: The Journal of Treatment & Prevention, 17*, 187–199.

Sagoe, D., Andreassen, C. S., & Pallesen, S. (2014). The aetiology and trajectory of anabolic-androgenic steroid use initiation: A systematic review and synthesis of qualitative research. *Substance Abuse Treatment, Prevention, and Policy, 9*, 27.

Smith, D., Hale, B., Rhea, D., Olrich, T., & Collier, K. (2009). Big, buff and dependent: Exercise dependence, muscle dysmorphia and steroid use in bodybuilding. In F. Columbus (Ed.), *Men and addictions*. New York: Nova Science.

Spence, J. C., McGannon, K. R., & Poon, P. (2005). The effect of exercise on global self-esteem: A quantitative review. *Journal of Sport & Exercise Psychology, 27*, 311–334.

Thiblin, I., Runeson, B., & Rajs, R. (1999). Anabolic androgenic steroids and suicide. *Annals of Clinical Psychiatry, 11*, 223–231.

Vassallo, M. J., & Olrich, T. W. (2010). Confidence by injection: Male users of anabolic steroids speak of increases in perceived confidence through anabolic steroid use. *International Journal of Sport and Exercise Psychology, 8*, 70–80.

Winett, R. A., & Carpinelli, R. N. (2001). Potential health-related benefits of resistance training. *Preventive Medicine: An International Journal Devoted to Practice and Theory, 33*, 503–513.

Wolke, D., & Sapouna, M. (2008). Big men feeling small: Childhood bullying experience, muscle dysmorphia and other mental health problems in bodybuilders. *Psychology of Sport and Exercise, 9*, 595–604.

4

Use of Drugs to Change Appearance in Girls and Female Adolescents

Jennifer O'Dea and Renata Leah Cinelli

The 'Appearance Culture' Among Adolescent Girls

In contemporary Western society a great deal of importance is placed on appearance, weight, shape, and beauty for women. The media is known to depict narrow appearance ideals that are not representative of the general population (Diedrichs et al. 2011), leaving many young girls failing to meet the prescribed 'standards'. Tiggemann (2011) describes the ideals as portraying women who are *young, tall, long-legged, large-eyed, moderately large-breasted, tanned but not too tanned, and clear-skinned women with usually White features* (p. 13). Diedrichs et al. (2011) participants' similarly stated ... *there is this stereotypical, blonde female with large*

J. O'Dea (✉)
Faculty of Education & Social Work, The University of Sydney, Sydney, NSW, 2006, Australia

R.L. Cinelli
Faculty of Education and Arts, Australian Catholic University, Victoria Pde, 250, 3002 East Melbourne, VIC, Australia

© The Editor(s) (if applicable) and The Author(s) 2016
M. Hall et al. (eds.), *Chemically Modified Bodies*,
DOI 10.1057/978-1-137-53535-1_4

breasts and the perfect body. No cellulite, and … she is quite slim. And girls aspire to be that … (p. 261). The old adage *what is beautiful is good* (Dion et al. 1972) and the stereotypes that physically attractive people *have it all* (Cash et al. 2004b), and are more sociable, friendly, warm, competent, and intelligent than less attractive people (Lorenzo et al. 2010), places physical appearance on the body modification agenda.

Further, the understanding that body weight and attractiveness is associated with positive attributes is often present even in very young girls. Research shows that girls as young as 3.5 years old selected thin or average dolls (over a fat doll) as being *pretty, helping others, having a best friend,* and being *smart* and *happy* (Worobey and Worobey 2014). Hence, it is no surprise that girls and adolescent females strive to meet these appearance ideals and experience a great deal of body dissatisfaction, low self-esteem, and poor body image when the ideals prove unachievable.

The body dissatisfaction experienced by young and adult women is well established as something that affects up to 80 % of women around the world (Forbes et al. 2012). This discontent is so widespread that it is considered 'normative' (Sabik et al. 2010; Tiggemann 2011), with research suggesting even pre-adolescent girls are engaging in appearance evaluation and experiencing dissatisfaction (Sinton and Birch 2006). Further, there is a high degree of focus placed on appearance among adolescent females, which is partly influenced by the media representations of females of the same age (Hargreaves and Tiggemann 2003). This results in a high degree of appearance investment.

Appearance, which encompasses but is not limited to, weight, shape, skin (e.g. tone/tan, smoothness/scarring or wrinkles, tattoos, and piercings) and facial features (e.g. eye colour), is often viewed as modifiable through 'appearance work'. This appearance work is defined as the use of clothing, cosmetics, dieting, exercise, hair care, and other similar behaviours and practices employed to maintain or alter one's appearance (Hurd Clarke and Korotchenko 2011). Engaging in behaviours for modification or maintenance of physical appearance, can include extreme dieting, supplement, or drug use (such as nutritional supplements, stimulants, smoking, laxative use, diuretics, diet pills, and tanning pills), and can be physically and mentally harmful to girls, particularly during puberty, a time of rapid physical and emotional change. Studies representing adolescent perspectives on aspects of appearance have shown that many adolescent females believe *it is important to be tanned all year long* (Tella et al. 2013) and that internalization of appearance ideals is common. For instance, many young women reported they would *like my body to look like the bodies of people in the media* or that *reading magazines makes me want to change my appearance* (Lawler and Nixon 2011). Studies have also shown that adolescent girls who are trying to look like women in the media are also more likely to use products to improve their appearance or strength (Field et al. 2005).

Appearance investment is distinct from, but related to, body satisfaction (Forand et al. 2010; Tiggemann 2004). Where body satisfaction is primarily a positive/negative evaluation of one's body or body parts, appearance investment relates to one's attitudes about the importance of appearance (Forand et al. 2010). A high level of appearance investment is associated with spending a great deal of time attending to, and/or attempting to maintain or enhance, their appearance (Cash et al. 2004a). Hence, those who have a high level of appearance investment are more likely to spend time on appearance work. The extent to which adolescent females are investing in their appearance has implications for their choices to engage in potentially harmful change strategies.

This chapter will explore the appearance behaviours that girls and adolescent females engage in with specific reference to drugs or substances used for the purpose of appearance modification, including physical appearance and weight and shape as a facet of appearance. Drugs used for this purpose will be examined and socioeconomic trends will be examined. Poly drug use will be examined and the chapter will conclude with implications for school-based education.

Defining and Outlining Drug Use for Appearance Enhancement

Appearance-enhancing drugs are often regarded in conjunction with performance-enhancing drugs. Hildebrandt and Lai (2011) more specifically define appearance- and performance-enhancing drugs (APEDs) as a wide range of substances used to alter one's outward appearance or improve one's ability to achieve or succeed in domains where performance is based on physical appearance and strength. (p. 314)

While there is a plethora of literature informing on APED use among males (see Chap. 2), such as anabolic steroids, there is less known about the appearance-enhancing substances used and reasons for substance use among females. Despite this, drug misuse (such as cigarettes, alcohol, and prescription substances) among adolescent girls has increased over the last two decades, and as such is gaining increasing attention (Kumpfer et al. 2008). The majority of the literature surrounding drugs or supplements used for appearance enhancement among adolescent females revolve around weight maintenance and modification, and more specifically, weight loss.

Reflective of the Western 'necessity' for young women to be thin, many young girls have developed their own 'effective' weight control programs, which are often extreme and include smoking, amphetamine use, diuretics, laxatives, and diet pills (Kumpfer et al. 2008; Grigg et al. 1996). Kumpfer and colleagues also discuss the 'Virginia Slims' effect promoted in an advertising campaign (for cigarettes) from over two decades ago, and how media campaigns such as this had an impact on drug use among adolescent females for reducing weight (see also Kumpfer et al. 1990). The concern regarding adolescent females and substance use for weight control is not new, with Grigg et al. (1996) reporting that over one-third of their adolescent female sample engaged in 'extreme' dieting methods such as using slimming tablets, laxatives, and cigarettes almost two decades ago. More recently, Pisetsky et al. (2008) provided further evidence of the use of substances for weight control among adolescent females in the USA. Adolescent females who reported disordered eating also reported higher rates of cigarette smoking (35.0 % versus 15.6 %), cocaine use (9.0 % versus 2.0 %), and steroid use (8.2 % versus 1.7 %) (Pisetsky et al. 2008). The trend towards higher substance use among adolescent females with disordered eating also included binge drinking, marijuana, methamphetamines, ecstasy, and hallucinogens.

Similarly, another study with adolescent females has found links between tanning bed use, concerns about weight, frequency of dieting to lose weight, smoking cigarettes, using laxatives or vomiting to control weight, binge drinking, using recreational drugs, and trying to look like women in the media (O'Riordan et al. 2006). These findings indicate that those young women who have concerns about their weight, shape, and appearance will often engage in more than one harmful behaviour in an effort to initiate change. Unfortunately, many of these change attempts are potentially health damaging. Some of the drugs and substances used by adolescent girls for appearance change and enhancement are further elaborated upon next.

Anabolic-Androgenic Steroids

Anabolic-androgenic steroids (AAS) are often used for increased lean muscle mass and strength, and a reduction in body fat, with side effects in women that can include acne, irregular menstrual cycles, depression, mood instability, organ damage, infertility, and breast atrophy (Committee on Gynecologic Practice 2011). Historically, greater use of AAS has been associated with athletes, but recent research suggests that AAS use is also a problem among non-athletes, particularly given the propensity of users to also be using other drugs or substances (Harmer 2010). Another study on adolescents purports that despite early findings, there is no difference in AAS use among athletes and non-athletes (Naylor et al. 2001).

Despite this, the reasons for use of AAS may vary between athletes and non-athletes. Bahrke and Yesalis (2004) explain that many athletes use AAS based on which sport they participate in: bodybuilders desire more lean mass and lower body fat, field athletes want the strength to 'out throw' their competitors, while swimmers and runners desire the ability to perform frequent, high-intensity workouts without physical breakdown. Beyond athletes, users of AAS often do so because they want to 'look good', which to some means being bigger or having a degree of muscularity (Bahrke and Yesalis 2004).

Usage among adolescents is known to be higher than usage among the general population (Dunn and White 2011), which is salient given the known potential side effects of steroid usage and the amount of physical development that takes place during adolescence. Within the adolescent population, literature confirms that steroid use among females is typically lower than that among males (Field et al. 2005; Eisenberg et al. 2012), with use among Australian adolescent females found to be around 1.2 % to 1.3 % (Dunn and White 2011; Handelsman and Gupta 1997). The prevalence of use among adolescent females around the world, reported at 0.8 % to 2.9 % in the USA (Hoffman et al. 2008; Miller et al. 2005; DiClemente et al. 2014); 0.6 % in Norway (Pallesen et al. 2006); and 2.8 % in Poland (Sas-Nowosielski 2006), contributes to the general consensus that use among non-athlete adolescent females is generally less than around 2.9 %. A more recent study found that among adolescent females, up to 4.5 % had used steroids in the previous 12 months, with usage reported as rarely, sometimes, or often (Eisenberg et al. 2012). This suggests there may have been an increase in usage, or at least higher rates of young women are experimenting with AAS usage, even if not being regular users.

Stimulant Drugs (Amphetamines, Ecstasy, and Cocaine)

Stimulant drugs such as amphetamines and cocaine have also been used among girls for weight loss (Pisetsky et al. 2008), despite the fact that they also carry the potential side effects of depression, anxiety, mood swings, paranoia, difficulty concentrating, suicidal ideation, and psychosis (Baker and Dawe 2005). Using stimulant drugs such as ecstasy, cocaine, and amphetamines to curb appetite and lose weight is known as 'instrumental use' (i.e. use based on the drug's effects for a purpose) (Boys et al. 2001). With knowledge of its appetite suppressant quality, studies have long reported that many female cocaine users name weight control as a primary motivator for use of the substance (Cochrane et al. 1998).

It is also suggested that many girls turn to 'club drugs' containing amphetamines to maintain the idealised image of the *happy, thin girl* (Kumpfer et al. 2008). Other studies have also confirmed that the reasons for use of harmful substances among young girls generally include concerns about weight and dieting (Pisetsky et al. 2008). A salient study with 16–22-year-olds investigated the perceived functions of drugs currently used among the cohort, and some of their reasons for use (Boys et al. 2001). A proportion of youths who had engaged in use of various substances more than once, reported use of certain drugs because they can *help you lose weight*. Specifically, 6 % of cocaine users, 23.1 % of amphetamine users, and 7 % of ecstasy users did so for the perceived weight-control properties (Boys et al. 2001). Despite this, research has shown that cocaine use may not actually reduce food intake, but rather just delay it, with higher levels of uncontrolled food intake reported among chronic cocaine users than healthy volunteers (Ersche et al. 2013).

While there are few studies that specifically examine the use of drugs such as amphetamines for the purpose of weight loss among adolescents, there are several publications that link substance abuse and eating disorders as comorbidities (Cochrane et al. 1998; Dennis and Pryor 2014). Wolfe and Maisto (2000) provide a review of literature that outlines a connection between subthreshold eating disorder symptomatology (e.g. bingeing, purging, restrained eating, and dysfunctional attitudes about weight and body shape) and substance use. Hence, often an increase in substance use occurs alongside an increase in disordered eating among high school and college students.

Considering these known links between eating and weight concerns and disturbance, comorbid drug use and abuse, and poor health outcomes, further research is needed to specifically examine the motivations behind drug use among adolescent girls.

Diet Pills, Slimming Pills, and Laxatives

The consumption of diet pills is often classified as an 'extreme' weight-control behaviour, with the primary intention being to lose weight or keep from gaining weight. Neumark-Sztainer et al. (2006) classified the use of diet pills as 'unhealthful' weight control, alongside cigarette smoking, food substitutes, laxatives, and diuretics. While some substances are used for their perceived appetite suppressant qualities, others are used because they assist in 'eliminating' or reducing what has been consumed.

For instance, diuretics are often used for weight control as they increase urine output, with the potential side effects of dizziness, dehydration, and hypertension (Franckowiak 2014).

Among adolescent females, 57.8 % were found to engage in at least one of these 'unhealthful' weight-control methods (Neumark-Sztainer et al. 2006). Another study showed diet pills were used without a doctors' advice by 11 % of the female adolescents for weight management (Lowry et al. 2002), while others reported diet products (including diet pills) were used by 7.7 % (Pisetsky et al. 2008) and 6 % (Wertheim et al. 1992) of adolescent females. Another study showed that of 1495 adolescent females, 7.8 % used diet pills and/or vomiting to control their weight in the past seven days (Middleman et al. 1998). Beyond diet pills, laxatives have also been used in the absence of doctors' advice by 4.8 % of the adolescent females in the US study (Lowry et al. 2002).

The following table presents a comparison of data on drug use for weight control by low, middle, and high SES status among male and female adolescents in Australia from a recent nationally representative study of 13,000 Australian schoolchildren (Table 4.1).

Results found an overall prevalence of diet pill and/or diuretic use of 2.0 % among females, as well as a significantly lower prevalence among same-aged males (1 %). Diet pill/diuretic abuse was more common in low SES males and low/middle SES females. Whilst laxative abuse for weight loss was similar among males and females respectively (1.2 and 1.3 %), the differences in SES were significant with laxative abuse more common in low SES males.

These new findings are difficult to explain, but they do suggest that social class plays some sort of role in the misuse and/or abuse of drugs for the enhancement of appearance associated with weight. In comparison to earlier studies from Australian adolescents, the prevalence of diet pill use appears to be lower than the early study of Wertheim et al. (1992) and similar to the early findings of O'Dea et al. (1996). While there is variance in the rates of use of these substances in the findings, it can be concluded that substance use for weight control has persisted among adolescent females over the past several decades and remains a salient area for health education and health promotion.

Table 4.1 Drug use for weight control in male and female Australian adolescents of low, middle, and high socioeconomic status in 2012

	Male (N = 3334)									Female (N = 3131)								
	Low SES (n = 321)		Middle SES (n = 2722)		High SES (n = 291)		Total (N = 3334)		χ^2	Low SES (n = 271)		Middle SES (n = 2595)		High SES (n = 265)		Total (N = 3131)		χ^2
	%	n	%	n	%	n	%	N		%	n	%	n	%	n	%	n	
Diuretics/diet pills	2.5	(8)	0.9	(25)	0.0	(0)	1.0	(33)	10.41*	2.6	(7)	2.1	(55)	0.8	(2)	2.0	(64)	12.14**
Laxatives	2.8	(9)	1.1	(29)	0.7	(2)	1.2	(40)	8.14*	1.8	(5)	1.5	(38)	0.8	(2)	1.3	(85)	1.20

Note. $*p < 0.05$, $**p < 0.01$, df = 1, Chi square = low and middle SES were more likely to use diuretics or slimming pills than the high SES

Cigarette Smoking

There is a plethora of literature from the past three decades outlining the links between body image and weight concerns, cigarette smoking, and smoking initiation among adolescents (Potter et al. 2004). Following the mention of the 'Virginia Slims' campaign (Kumpfer et al. 2008), cigarettes have also long been associated with weight loss or weight maintenance. In a large study (N = 15,349) of high school students in the USA, over 60 % reported trying to either maintain their current weight or lose weight. Trying to lose weight was associated with cigarette smoking among the girls, with 39 % of the girls who reported smoking also reporting trying to lose weight (Lowry et al. 2002). That same study also found that current smoking was associated with using diet pills and vomiting or using laxatives for weight control.

In another study with 1560 sixth- and seventh-grade students in Boston and Austin, USA, Gortmaker (2001) found that the relation between dieting frequency and smoking initiation was significant among the adolescent females, while Potter et al. (2004) also found dieting behaviours, disordered eating symptoms, and weight concerns had a positive relationship with smoking. These studies all provide support for the links between desired weight loss and smoking as an unhealthy weight control method, and indicate this is an important area to target in health education for adolescent females.

The following table presents a comparison of data on smoking to reduce appetite and to lose weight by low, middle, and high SES status among male and female adolescents in Australia from a recent nationally representative study of 13,000 Australian schoolchildren (Table 4.2).

The results in Table 4.2, despite not reaching statistical significance, suggest that low SES males are more likely than their middle or high SES counterparts to use cigarette smoking as a form of weight control. A similar graded trend is also apparent among adolescent females with low SES females reporting smoking to reduce appetite and to lose weight three times more frequently than high SES girls.

Table 4.2 Smoking for weight loss in male and female Australian adolescents of low, middle, and high socioeconomic status in 2012

	Male (N = 3343)									Female (N = 3124)								
	Low SES (n = 321)		Middle SES (n = 2731)		High SES (n = 291)		Total (N = 3343)		χ^2	Low SES (n = 272)		Middle SES (n = 2587)		High SES (n = 265)		Total (N = 3131)		χ^2
	%	n	%	n	%	n	%	n		%	n	%	n	%	n	%	n	
Smoking to reduce appetite and to lose weight	1.9	(6)	1.4	(39)	0.3	(1)	1.4	(46)	2.30	3.7	(10)	2.6	(66)	1.1	(3)	2.5	(79)	3.56

Chi square = low and middle SES were more likely to smoke for weight loss than the high SES

Whilst these results should be considered with caution in light of the fact that these trends were not statistically significant, they should be further investigated to determine whether the trend is replicable, or simply occurs due to chance. SES is certainly linked to the prevalence of overweight and obesity in children and adolescents in Australia, and therefore, the trend for greater weight control may reflect this. In addition, smoking prevalence is graded by SES, so the trend may simply reflect general population smoking patterns rather than smoking for deliberate weight control. Further research should examine this topic, possibly using qualitative methods to tease out these potential trends.

Nutritional Supplements

Franckowiak (2014) discussed the increased pressures that young people are facing in modern society, to look a certain way and to stand out and succeed. As such, the use of nutritional supplements such as protein or creatine is increasing among adolescents, particularly among those who desire improvement in sports performance and physical appearance (Lucidi et al. 2008). Eisenberg et al. (2012) examined the use of numerous muscle-enhancing substances among adolescents, and reported that the girls, who were most concerned with weight control, were more likely to use protein powders and shakes than other substances. Specifically, over 20 % of the 1486 adolescent females in the study reported having used protein powders or shakes in the previous 12 months. Similarly, in the study by Field and her colleagues (2005), protein powders and shakes were the products most often used to improve appearance, and had been used by 8 % of girls throughout the previous year.

Beyond this, recent prevalence data are lacking about the use of creatine among children and adolescents. In a 2005 sample of 6212 American girls (aged 9–14), only small proportions reported weekly creatine (0.1 %) or protein (shakes or powder) (1.4 %) use for improvement of physical appearance or for gaining weight, strength, or muscle mass (Field et al. 2005). The use of nutritional supplements, such as creatine and amino acids (Bell et al. 2004), have also been reported as prevalent among adolescents, especially those who seek to improve their performance and physical appearance (Calfee and Fadale 2006; Metzl et al. 2001; Lucidi et al. 2008; O'Dea 2003).

While athletes use doping substances primarily to improve their performance, adolescent non-athletes do so mainly to enhance their physical appearance (Lucidi et al. 2008). In the study by Lucidi and colleagues, just over 2 % of the participating adolescents reported to have used at least one doping substance in the previous three months, whereas nearly 15 % of them reported to have used at least one nutritional supplement during the same period (Lucidi et al. 2008).

Beyond the non-athlete specific samples discussed, protein powder or protein supplements have been used for weight gain or increasing muscle mass among female athletes around the world, albeit to a lesser extent than among their male counterparts (see Chap. 2). For instance, usage was reported among 4 % of Singaporean adolescent female athletes (versus 20 % among males) (Slater et al. 2003), and among 6 % of Canadian female athletes (versus 11 % of males) (Erdman et al. 2007). In Canada, the use of 'extra protein' (27 %) was much more prevalent than the use of steroids (2.8 %) (Melia et al. 1996).

While the use of extra protein or other nutritional substances is common practice for many young athletes, use of nutritional substances has been associated with the 'gateway hypotheses', where nutritional supplement use may lead to the use of doping substances. Up to 40 % of female athletes under 18 have reported being nutritional supplement users (Petroczi and Naughton 2008), with that proportion increasing in young adult athletes. Another study found that athletes who used nutritional supplements (compared with non-users) were more willing to take a substance that would give them a more athletic body and change their weight in a desirable direction (either losing or gaining weight) based on their chosen sport (Backhouse et al. 2013).

The aforementioned findings indicate that supplement use is relatively common among adolescent females, regardless of athlete status, particularly when contrasted with doping substances. This has implications for the nutrition, body image, and physical education of young adolescent females.

Tanning Products

Beyond weight control, Tiggemann's (2011) descriptions of the ideal woman represented in modern mainstream media, including being *tanned* and *clear-skinned*, also reflect the numerous supplements and products which are available and used among young women to target these specific aspects of appearance. For example, the market provides ingestible tablets that promote tanning (e.g. *Tanamins* or *tanning pills*) or minerals that are marketed for the promotion of clear skin and shiny hair (e.g. *silica tablets*). The substances used could be viewed as existing on a continuum, with readily available, over-the-counter, legal drugs at one end (such as cigarettes, laxatives, some diet pills, tanning pills), and prescription and illicit drugs at the other (such as cocaine and other amphetamines or stimulants, anabolic steroids). In addition, access to a wide range of supplements and drugs is rarely an issue for potential users as a broad range of drugs used for enhancement purposes are often obtainable via illicit markets and online (Breindahl et al. 2015; Field et al. 2005). Use, and/or misuse of legal and illegal substances, regardless of access and legality, can have varying degrees of physiological implications or side effects for users.

The concept that standards of beauty, appearance, and social body ideals are entrenched in culture and society is not new. Considering the global depth and variety of culture, it is unsurprising that the practices adolescent females engage in to modify or change appearance, would vary based on differing cultural mores, desired outcomes, and contexts. Different cultures are known to place stronger emphasis on different components of appearance, with some emphasising thinness, others muscularity and strength, and others skin tone and appearance.

Skin tone is one facet of appearance where the desire and practices can vary greatly around the world. A study of French adolescents (N = 713) indicated that over half of the cohort believed it was important to be tanned over summer, many females believed it was important to be tanned all year long, and females were more likely than males to have used tanning pills (Tella et al. 2013). In contrast, an earlier study showed that a *minority* of females in Japan desired tanned skin, and of those who did, the majority wished to recover their normal skin tone following summer (Fukuda and Naganuma 1997).

In Western societies, there has been an increase in the level of products sold and used to increase skin pigmentation for cosmetic reasons (Breindahl et al. 2015). In the French study, 1 % of female adolescents reported using tanning pills (Tella et al. 2013), which is likely to be increasing alongside other sunless tanning products owing to the known harmful effects of solar and artificial ultraviolet (UV) radiation (Chisvert et al. 2011; O'Riordan et al. 2006). While there is little published literature surrounding the prevalence of tanning pill use among adolescent females, it is likely that usage is reflected in cultural values. For instance, value placed on tanning or darker skin is particularly Western, since having a tan in some countries (for instance some Asian countries) is traditionally associated with being a field worker and of a lower social class. Fukuda and Naganuma (1997) reported that only 37 % of Japanese women wanted a tan, compared with 100 % of American women who desired tanned skin on either their face, body, or both. Hence, despite the lack of published data, it is likely that the desire for tanned skin and usage of tanning pills in countries such as Australia, Europe, and the USA is higher than in other non-Western countries. The particularly high rates of skin cancer in Australia, Europe and the USA (Diepgen and Mahler 2002) contrast with the use of skin-whitening products such as 'Bihaku' in Japan and other Asian countries. This contrasting behaviour provides further evidence of how the value placed on tanned skin as 'beautiful' is often culturally based.

Implications for School-Based Education

The issue of drug and substance use to change appearance in girls needs to be further studied in order to understand any potentially unhealthy or risky behaviour and to plan health education around this topic. The reasons for drug use among girls suggest a desire for general features of the Western ideals including slimness, athletic appearance, sports performance, and tanning. The results of this recent literature review suggest that there has been a shift in consumption patterns among adolescent girls, who now appear to use drugs and other supplements independently of any parental direction. For example, a seminal, large American study Ervin et al. (1999) found that nutritional supplementation was more likely to occur among females, children aged 1–5 years, Caucasians, those with a higher income, higher educational status, and greater self-reported health status. More recently, girls and older adolescent females have reported accessing and consuming dieting pills, diuretics, laxatives, cocaine, amphetamines, or stimulants for weight control and nutritional supplements such as amino acids, protein, and creatine, as well as anabolic steroids for improved sports performance and athletic appearance (Dunn and White 2011; Eisenberg et al. 2012; Pisetsky et al. 2008; Lucidi et al. 2008; Lowry et al. 2002).

The perceptions of parents, teachers, and sports coaches are important to the understanding of appearance-enhancing drugs. This is particularly salient in school-based education about this issue, because research suggests that mothers and stakeholders are likely to influence adolescent behaviour by supplying the supplements to children and adolescents. For example, the reasons for nutritional supplementation reported by children and adolescents in an Australian study (O'Dea 2003) varied according to the type of supplement being consumed. Vitamin and mineral supplements and herbal supplements were taken by adolescents to promote better health, to prevent illnesses such as the common cold and because they were given to participants by their mother. It is also likely that diet pills and diuretics are sourced by girls via drugs that have been prescribed for their mothers.

The association with sports performance and appearance is also relevant to further study, as early studies of adolescent athletes (Douglas and Douglas 1984; Carruth and Goldberg 1990; Sobal and Marquart 1994; Haymes 1991) show that a better sports performance is expected by nutritional supplement users. More recent studies confirm these original findings, with girls continuing to use nutritional supplements for the purpose of body change or enhanced performance (Eisenberg et al. 2012; Lucidi et al. 2008; Calfee and Fadale 2006).

Similar findings have been reported in a study of male and female adolescents in Australia which aimed to obtain rich qualitative data about the type of nutritional supplements and drinks consumed by adolescents, and the reasons for their consumption, with particular emphasis on the perceived benefits of nutritional supplementation (O'Dea 2003). Participants reported consuming sports drinks, vitamin and mineral supplements, energy drinks, herbal supplements, guarana, creatine, high-protein milk supplements, and coenzyme Q10. Reasons for supplement use included perceived short-term health benefits, prevention of illness, improved immunity, parental supply of supplements, taste, energy boost, better sports performance and to rectify a poor diet. Results suggest that some adolescents consume nutritional supplements, sports drinks, and energy drinks for their perceived physiological benefits, and that they may not be aware of any potential risks.

Use of Health Education Theory for School-Based Prevention Programs

The use of health education theory can help to improve our understanding of the nutritional supplementation practices and drug use of adolescents for appearance-enhancing purposes. Health education theory generally states that a person's behaviour and cognitions affect future behaviour, and that in order to improve adolescents' health behaviours, we need to understand the many factors which influence behaviour and the complex interactions between such variables (Bandura 1986; Glanz et al. 2002).

An important theoretical model on which to base school education relating to education about nutritional supplementation practices and drug use of adolescents for appearance-enhancing purposes is the *Health Belief Model* (Ajzen 1991) which consists of four constructs representing the perceived threats and net benefits including—perceived susceptibility, perceived severity, perceived benefits, and perceived barriers. Use of such health education theory to prevent health risks in girls would involve students exploring these facets of their risk taking behaviours.

Another relevant health education theory includes *Social Cognitive Theory* (Bandura 1986) which posits that many factors interact to affect behaviour, including actual behaviour, personal factors (including cognitions), and environmental influences. An understanding of the many factors which affect girls' nutritional supplementation and drug use practices, both in research and within educational discussions, will help to educate young people better about the risks and benefits of such behaviours. For example, by utilising the theory in order to prevent health-damaging outcomes of drug taking such as the potential side effects of steroids, diuretics or tanning pills, educators first need to understand the perceived benefits, risks, individual perceptions, self-efficacy, and environmental factors which drive the consumption of such products among adolescent girls. Such information can be derived from both qualitative and quantitative research studies as well as in-class critical discussions with students.

The findings outlined in this chapter have a wide range of implications for school-based health education, health promotion, and drug prevention programs. Popular programs that have aimed to reduce body dissatisfaction among young females have included body image prevention programming that focuses on discussions about the influence of peers and the media, and were designed to prevent weight loss behaviours. A new focus for girls might be to allow students to examine how and why girls engage in risk taking to improve their appearance and how they implement weight change behaviours for the purposes of gaining strength and improving sports performance. Such body image prevention programmes should focus on the primary drivers for girls engaging in drug use for weight and appearance change behaviours. Similarly, interventions to prevent the use of steroids among girls should essentially target body dissatisfaction.

One new educational program for boys is the Athletes Training and Learning to Avoid Steroids [ATLAS] program (Goldberg et al. 2000) which represents best practice in the prevention of anabolic steroid use among male high school athletes in the USA. The most recent trial involved 3207 male adolescent football players in the USA, who participated in a program that included nutrition information, role plays of drug refusal and discussion of alternate strategies to improve performance. This theory-based session was supported by a weights session in the gym each week. Classes were conducted by coaches and trainers, and achieved significant increases in self-esteem, knowledge about the harmful effects of steroids, and attitudes towards media advertisements (Goldberg et al.

2000). Intentions to use anabolic steroids were also lowered at post-test and one-year follow-up. It is suggested that this sort of content could make body image programming more relevant for young females who are at risk of drug use for appearance enhancement. Teaching and learning materials could include factual information about the potential harmful effects of using supplements and other body-enhancing drugs in the same way that we discuss the dangers of dieting. Programs could then provide information about safe and effective ways to achieve body satisfaction, self-acceptance, body-esteem, media literacy, healthy weight control, and a safe artificial tan. Such educational programs should include the inclusion of specific types of physical activity, such as those in recent programs aimed at girls (Burgess et al. 2006; Neumark-Sztainer et al. 2010).

This research suggests that, due to the relationship between body image, use of supplements, and attitudes towards the use of drugs in sport, educators should incorporate school-based health education approaches that incorporate the prevention of drug use for appearance with interventions to prevent body dissatisfaction. Both broad-ranging and targeted prevention approaches are likely to improve the physical and psychological health of girls and boys in the short term, as they are less likely to suffer from body dissatisfaction, and the negative side effects of using drugs, supplements, and anabolic steroids.

Summary

While there is ample research outlining that concern with muscle definition and media images may lead young people to use unhealthful products to achieve a more desired physique (Field et al. 2005), there are also suggestions of what might be effective in addressing and preventing concerns, and hence reducing the unhealthful product use. In their review, Kumpfer et al. (2008) discussed the early use of social resistance assertiveness training which could be useful considering the known impact of peers on body image and associated change behaviours. In reviewing programs aimed at reducing initiation and use of certain drugs, Kumpfer et al. (2008) outlined the importance of implementing programs to target young adolescents, explicitly teaching social resistance skills, and understanding the negative influence of social norms. Other prevention strategies found to be beneficial include family bonding, parental supervision, and communication. Further, interventions to promote healthy weight management among adolescents should discourage reliance on extreme and potentially dangerous weight-control methods, especially among females and overweight adolescents (Lowry et al. 2002).

The apparent willingness of adolescents to use a supplement that may harm their health or shorten their life highlights the need for greater involvement of teachers, coaches, and physicians to provide continued education on the risks and benefits associated with nutritional supplementation and AAS use (Hoffman et al. 2008). Adolescents also seemed willing to take more risks with supplements to achieve their fitness or athletic goals, even if these risks reduced health or caused premature death (Kumpfer et al. 1990).

Further it is important to contextualise the willingness of young people to take health risks, and understand the impact feedback from peers and others can have on the health perceptions and choices of young women. Even positive feedback about weight and body shape can have a negative impact on the body image of young women, as positive comments often serve to remind young people that they are being evaluated on their looks, appearance and body (Nowell and Ricciardelli 2008). Care must therefore be taken when educating young people, with an emphasis placed on healthy eating and exercise as opposed to weight, shape, and appearance.

References

Ajzen, I. (1991). The theory of planned behavior. *Organizational Behavior and Human Decision Processes, 50*, 179–211.

Austin, S. B., & Gortmaker, S. L. (2001). Dieting and smoking initiation in early adolescent girls and boys: A prospective study. *American Journal of Public Health, 91*, 446.

Backhouse, S., Whitaker, L., & Petróczi, A. (2013). Gateway to doping? Supplement use in the context of preferred competitive situations, doping attitude, beliefs, and norms. *Scandinavian Journal of Medicine and Science in Sports, 23*, 244–252.

Bahrke, M. S., & Yesalis, C. E. (2004). Abuse of anabolic androgenic steroids and related substances in sport and exercise. *Current Opinion in Pharmacology, 4*, 614–620.

Baker, A., & Dawe, S. (2005). Amphetamine use and co-occurring psychological problems: Review of the literature and implications for treatment. *Australian Psychologist, 40*, 88–95.

Bandura, A. (1986). *Social foundations of thought and action*. Englewood Cliffs, NJ: Prentice-Hall.

Bell, A., Dorsch, K. D., Mccreary, D. R., & Hovey, R. (2004). A look at nutritional supplement use in adolescents. *Journal of Adolescent Health, 34*(6), 508–516.

Boys, A., Marsden, J., & Strang, J. (2001). Understanding reasons for drug use amongst young people: A functional perspective. *Health Education Research, 16*, 457–469.

Breindahl, T., Evans-Brown, M., Hindersson, P., McVeigh, J., Bellis, M., Stensballe, A., et al. (2015). Identification and characterization by LC-UV-MS/MS of melanotan II skin-tanning products sold illegally on the Internet. *Drug Testing and Analysis, 7*, 164–172.

Burgess, G., Grogan, S., & Burwitz, L. (2006). Effects of a 6-week aerobic dance intervention on body image and physical self-perceptions in adolescent girls. *Body Image, 3*, 57–66.

Calfee, R., & Fadale, P. (2006). Popular ergogenic drugs and supplements in young athletes. *Pediatrics, 117*, e577–e589.

Carruth, B. R., & Goldberg, D. L. (1990). Nutritional issues of adolescents: Athletics and the body image mania. *The Journal of Early Adolescence, 10*, 122–140.

Cash, T. F., Jakatdar, T. A., & Williams, E. F. (2004a). The body image quality of life inventory: Further validation with college men and women. *Body Image, 1*, 279–287.

Cash, T. F., Melnyk, S. E., & Hrabosky, J. I. (2004b). The assessment of body image investment: An extensive revision of the appearance schemas inventory. *International Journal of Eating Disorders, 35*, 305–316.

Chisvert, A., Balaguer, A., & Salvador, A. (2007). Tanning and whitening agents in cosmetics. Regulatory aspects and analytical methods. In A. Salvador & A. Chisvert (Eds.), *Analysis of Cosmetic Products* (pp. 128–140). Amsterdam: Elsevier.

Cochrane, C., Malcolm, R., & Brewerton, T. (1998). The role of weight control as a motivation for cocaine abuse. *Addictive Behaviors, 23*, 201–207.

Committee on Gynecologic Practice. (2011). Performance enhancing anabolic steroid abuse in women. Committee Opinion No. 484, *American College of Obstetricians and Gynecologists*, 117, 1016–1018.

Dennis, A., & Pryor, T. (2014). Introduction to substance use disorders for the eating disorder specialist. In T. D. Brewerton & A. Baker Dennis (Eds.), *Eating disorders, addictions and substance use disorders*. Berlin Heidelberg: Springer.

DiClemente, R., Jackson, J., Hertzberg, V., & Seth, P. (2014). Steroid use, health risk behaviors and adverse health indicators among us high school students. *Family Medicine & Medical Science Research, 3*, 2.

Diedrichs, P. C., Lee, C., & Kelly, M. (2011). Seeing the beauty in everyday people: A qualitative study of young Australians' opinions on body image, the mass media and models. *Body Image, 8*, 259–266.

Diepgen, T. L., & Mahler, V. (2002). The epidemiology of skin cancer. *British Journal of Dermatology, 146*, 1–6.

Dion, K., Berscheid, E., & Walster, E. (1972). What is beautiful is good. *Journal of Personality and Social Psychology, 24*, 285.

Douglas, P. D., & Douglas, J. G. (1984). Nutrition knowledge and food practices of high school athletes. *Journal of the American Dietetic Association, 84*, 1198–1202.

Dunn, M., & White, V. (2011). The epidemiology of anabolic–androgenic steroid use among Australian secondary school students. *Journal of Science and Medicine in Sport, 14*, 10–14.

Eisenberg, M. E., Wall, M., & Neumark-Sztainer, D. (2012). Muscle-enhancing behaviors among adolescent girls and boys. *Pediatrics, 130*, 1019–1026.

Erdman, K. A., Fung, T. S., Doyle-Baker, P. K., Verhoef, M. J., & Reimer, R. A. (2007). Dietary supplementation of high-performance Canadian athletes by age and gender. *Clinical Journal of Sport Medicine, 17*, 458–464.

Ersche, K. D., Stochl, J., Woodward, J. M., & Fletcher, P. C. (2013). The skinny on cocaine: Insights into eating behavior and body weight in cocaine-dependent men. *Appetite, 71*, 75–80.

Ervin, R. B., Wright, J. D., & Kennedy-Stephenson, J. (1999). Use of dietary supplements in the United States. 1988–94, *Vital and Health Statistics. Series 11, Data from the National Health Survey*, i–iii, 1–14.

Field, A. E., Austin, S. B., Camargo, C. A., Taylor, C. B., Striegel-Moore, R. H., Loud, K. J., et al. (2005). Exposure to the mass media, body shape concerns, and use of supplements to improve weight and shape among male and female adolescents. *Pediatrics, 116*, e214–e220.

Forand, N. R., Gunthert, K. C., German, R. E., & Wenze, S. J. (2010). Appearance investment and everyday interpersonal functioning: An experience sampling study. *Psychology of Women Quarterly, 34*, 380–393.

Forbes, G. B., Jung, J., Vaamonde, J. D., Omar, A., Paris, L., & Formiga, N. S. (2012). Body dissatisfaction and disordered eating in three cultures: Argentina, Brazil, and the U.S. *Sex Roles, 66*, 677–694.

Franckowiak, B. (2014). Performance-enhancing drugs and the high school athlete. *NASN School Nurse, 30*(4), 214–216.

Fukuda, M., & Naganuma, M. (1997). The Sunscreen industry in Japan: Past, present and future. In N. J. Lowe, N. A. Shaath, & M. A. Pathak (Eds.), *Sunscreens: Development, evaluation and regulatory aspects* (pp. 241–259). New York: Marcel Dekker.

Glanz, K., Rimer, B. K., & Lewis, F. M. (Eds.) (2002). *Health behavior and health education: Theory, research, and practice* (3rd ed.). San Francisco: Jossey-Bass.

Goldberg, L., MacKinnon, D. P., Elliott, D. L., Moe, E. L., Clarke, G., & Cheong, J. (2000). The adolescents training and learning to avoid steroids program. *Archives of Pediatric and Adolescent Medicine, 154*, 322–338.

Grigg, M., Bowman, J., & Redman, S. (1996). Disordered eating and unhealthy weight reduction practices among adolescent females. *Preventive Medicine, 25*, 748–756.

Handelsman, D., & Gupta, L. (1997). Prevalence and risk factors for anabolic-androgenic steroid abuse in Australian high school students. *International Journal of Andrology, 20*, 159–164.

Hargreaves, D., & Tiggemann, M. (2003). The effect of "thin ideal" television commercials on body dissatisfaction and schema activation during early adolescence. *Journal of Youth and Adolescence, 32*, 367–373.

Harmer, P. A. (2010). Anabolic-androgenic steroid use among young male and female athletes: Is the game to blame? *British Journal of Sports Medicine, 44*, 26–31.

Haymes, E. M. (1991). Vitamin and mineral supplementation to athletes. *International Journal of Sport Nutrition, 1*, 146–169.

Hildebrandt, T., & Lai, J. (2011). Body image and appearance-and performance-enhancing drug use. In T. Cash & L. Smolak (Eds.), *Body image: A handbook of science, practice, and prevention* (pp. 314–320). New York: The Guilford Press.

Hoffman, J. R., Faigenbaum, A. D., Ratamess, N. A., Ross, R., Kang, J., & Tenenbaum, G. (2008). Nutritional supplementation and anabolic steroid use in adolescents. *Medicine and Science in Sports and Exercise, 40*, 15–24.

Hurd Clarke, L., & Korotchenko, A. (2011). Aging and the body: A review. *Canadian Journal on Aging, 30*, 495–510.

Kumpfer, K. L., Prazza, A. H., & Whiteside, H. O. (1990). Etiology of alcohol and other drug problems: Nature vs nurture. In R. C. Engs (Ed.), *Women: Alcohol and other drugs*. Dubuque, IA: Kendall Hunt Publishing Co.

Kumpfer, K. L., Smith, P., & Summerhays, J. F. (2008). A wakeup call to the prevention field: Are prevention programs for substance use effective for girls? *Substance Use & Misuse, 43*, 978–1001.

Lawler, M., & Nixon, E. (2011). Body dissatisfaction among adolescent boys and girls: The effects of body mass, peer appearance culture and internalization of appearance ideals. *Journal of Youth and Adolescence, 40*, 59–71.

Lorenzo, G. L., Biesanz, J. C., & Human, L. J. (2010). What is beautiful is good and more accurately understood physical attractiveness and accuracy in first impressions of personality. *Psychological Science, 21*, 1777–1782.

Lowry, R., Galuska, D. A., Fulton, J. E., Wechsler, H., & Kann, L. (2002). Weight management goals and practices among U.S. high school students: Associations with physical activity, diet, and smoking. *Journal of Adolescent Health, 31*, 133–144.

Lucidi, F., Zelli, A., Mallia, L., Grano, C., Russo, P. M., & Violani, C. (2008). The social-cognitive mechanisms regulating adolescents' use of doping substances. *Journal of Sports Sciences, 26*, 447–456.

Melia, P., Pipe, A., & Greenberg, L. (1996). The use of anabolic-androgenic steroids by Canadian students. *Clinical Journal of Sport Medicine, 6*, 9–14.

Metzl, J. D., Small, E., Levine, S. R., & Gershel, J. C. (2001). Creatine use among young athletes. *Pediatrics, 108*, 421–425.

Middleman, A. B., Vazquez, I., & Durant, R. H. (1998). Eating patterns, physical activity, and attempts to change weight among adolescents. *Journal of Adolescent Health, 22*, 37–42.

Miller, K. E., Hoffman, J. H., Barnes, G. M., Sabo, D., Melnick, M. J., & Farrell, M. P. (2005). Adolescent anabolic steroid use, gender, physical activity, and other problem behaviors. *Substance Use & Misuse, 40*, 1637–1657.

Naylor, A. H., Gardner, D., & Zaichkowsky, L. (2001). Drug use patterns among high school athletes and nonathletes. *Adolescence, 36*, 627–639.

Neumark-Sztainer, D., Friend, S. E., Flattum, C. F., Hannan, P. J., Story, M., Bauer, K. W., et al. (2010). New moves-preventing weight-related problems in adolescent girls: A group-randomised study. *American Journal of Preventive Medicine, 39*, 421–432.

Neumark-Sztainer, D., Wall, M., Guo, J., Story, M., Haines, J., & Eisenberg, M. (2006). Obesity, disordered eating, and eating disorders in a longitudinal study of adolescents: How do dieters fare 5 years later? *Journal of the American Dietetic Association, 106*, 559–568.

Nowell, C., & Ricciardelli, L. A. (2008). Appearance-based comments, body dissatisfaction and drive for muscularity in males. *Body Image, 5*, 337–345.

O'Dea, J., Abraham, S., & Heard, R. (1996). Food habits, body image and weight control practices of young male and female adolescents. *Australian Journal of Nutrition and Dietetics, 52*, 32–38.

O'Dea, J. A. (2003). Consumption of nutritional supplements among adolescents: Usage and perceived benefits. *Health Education Research, 18*, 98–107.

O'Riordan, D., Field, A., Geller, A., Brooks, D., Aweh, G., Colditz, G., et al. (2006). Frequent tanning bed use, weight concerns, and other health risk behaviors in adolescent females (United States). *Cancer Causes & Control, 17*, 679–686.

Pallesen, S., Jøsendal, O., Johnsen, B.-H., Larsen, S., & Molde, H. (2006). Anabolic steroid use in high school students. *Substance Use & Misuse, 41*, 1705–1717.

Petroczi, A., & Naughton, D. (2008). The age-gender-status profile of high performing athletes in the UK taking nutritional supplements: Lessons for the future. *Journal of the International Society of Sports Nutrition, 5*, 1–8.

Pisetsky, E. M., May Chao, Y., Dierker, L. C., May, A. M., & Striegel-Moore, R. H. (2008). Disordered eating and substance use in high-school students: Results from the Youth Risk Behavior Surveillance System. *International Journal of Eating Disorders, 41*, 464–470.

Potter, B. K., Pederson, L. L., Chan, S. S. H., Aubut, J.-A. L., & Koval, J. J. (2004). Does a relationship exist between body weight, concerns about weight, and smoking among adolescents? An integration of the literature with an emphasis on gender. *Nicotine & Tobacco Research, 6*, 397–425.

Sabik, N. J., Cole, E. R., & Ward, L. m. (2010). Are all minority women equally buffered from negative body image? Intra-ethnic moderators of the buffering hypothesis. *Psychology of Women Quarterly, 34*, 139–151.

Sas-Nowosielski, K. (2006). The abuse of anabolic-androgenic steroids by Polish school-aged adolescents. *Biology of Sport, 23*, 225.

Sinton, M., & Birch, L. (2006). Individual and sociocultural influences on preadolescent girls' appearance schemas and body dissatisfaction. *Journal of Youth and Adolescence, 35*, 157–167.

Slater, G., Tan, B., & Teh, K. C. (2003). Dietary supplementation practices of Singaporean athletes. *International Journal of Sport Nutrition and Exercise Metabolism, 13*, 320–332.

Sobal, J., & Marquart, L. F. (1994). Vitamin/mineral supplement use among high school athletes. *Adolescence, 29*(116), 835–843.

Tella, E., Beauchet, A., Vouldoukis, I., Séi, J. F., Beaulieu, P., Sigal, M. L., et al. (2013). French teenagers and artificial tanning. *Journal of the European Academy of Dermatology and Venereology, 27*, e428–e432.

Tiggemann, M. (2004). Body image across the adult lifespan: Stability and change. *Body Image, 1*, 29–41.

Tiggemann, M. (2011). Sociocultural perspectives on human appearance and body image. In T. F. Cash & L. Smolak (Eds.), *Body image: A handbook of science, practice, and prevention* (2nd ed.). New York: The Guilford Press.

Wertheim, E. H., Paxton, S. J., Maude, D., Szmukler, G. I., Gibbons, K., & Hillier, L. (1992). Psychosocial predictors of weight loss behaviors and binge eating in adolescent girls and boys. *International Journal of Eating Disorders, 12*, 151–160.

Wolfe, W. L., & Maisto, S. A. (2000). The relationship between eating disorders and substance use: Moving beyond co-prevalence research. *Clinical Psychology Review, 20*, 617–631.

Worobey, J., & Worobey, H. S. (2014). Body-size stigmatization by preschool girls: In a doll's world, it is good to be "Barbie". *Body Image, 11*, 171–174.

Part II

Non-prescription Substances

5

Caffeine Misuse and Weight Loss

Carla E. Ramacciotti, Elisabetta Coli,
and Annalisa Burgalassi

Mechanism of Action

Caffeine is a xanthine alkaloid compound that acts in the central nervous system as a non-selective adenosine receptor antagonist, and its main effects are as a psychostimulant from low to moderate doses it increases alertness and/or attention and reduces fatigue. It has been reported that caffeine, similar to other psychoactive compounds, when used chronically may induce a clinical dependence syndrome, and may provoke withdrawal symptoms, such as transient cognitive impairment and dysphoria,

---

C.E. Ramacciotti (✉)
Department of Clinical and Experimental Psichiatry, University of Pisa
Via Savi 10, 56126, Pisa, Italy

E. Coli
Department of Mental Health, Azienda USL Toscana Centro,
National Health Service, Italy

A. Burgalassi
Azienda USL Toscana Centro, National Health Service, Italy

© The Editor(s) (if applicable) and The Author(s) 2016
M. Hall et al. (eds.), *Chemically Modified Bodies*,
DOI 10.1057/978-1-137-53535-1_5

especially when its discontinuation is abrupt (Strain et al. 1994; Hughes et al. 1998; Thong et al. 2002). Several studies suggest caffeine has an influence on glucose tolerance and insulin sensitivity: ingestion of caffeine by lean persons before an oral-glucose-tolerance test resulted in a greater insulin response and no decrease in the glucose response; furthermore, acute caffeine ingestion significantly dampened whole-body insulin sensitivity in obese, nondiabetic persons (Graham et al. 2001; Thong and Graham 2002a; Petrie et al. 2004). Studies using hyperinsulinemic euglycemic clamps have confirmed that caffeine ingestion reduces whole-body glucose disposal by 15–30 % and glucose uptake in the leg muscle by 50 % (Greer et al. 2001; Keijzers et al. 2002; Thong et al. 2002). Although we know that skeletal muscle is the major tissue that becomes insulin-insensitive after caffeine ingestion, the mechanism of action is uncertain. Although many potential mechanisms exist, considerable evidence indicates that physiologic concentrations of caffeine antagonize adenosine receptors both in skeletal muscle and in the central nervous system, with the latter resulting in an increase in sympathetic activity (Vergauwen et al. 1994; Han et al. 1998; Fredholm 1998; Graham 2001; Thong and Graham 2002a, b).

Potential of Abuse

Because of the widespread use of caffeine and its known potent physiological effects, caffeine has long been the subject of research in psychological-related studies: caffeine ingestion and coffee drinking have been investigated with regard to the degree that this habit results in tolerance and withdrawal effects. These studies look beyond the obvious social implications and psychic dependence of coffee consumption which may be related to the "first cup of coffee to wake me up" or "the coffee break" or to its association with smoking. In the latter case, note that coffee drinkers took more nicotine when deprived of coffee (Bolton and Null 1981). Several human studies and one animal experiment suggest that physical dependence substantially potentiates the reinforcing effects of caffeine. Other human and animal studies indicate that there may be substantial differences between individual subjects in the reinforcing effects of caffeine. An important challenge for future human and animal drug self-administration research will be to delineate more precisely the conditions under which caffeine does and does not serve reliably as reinforcement (Griffiths and Woodson 1988).

Caffeine has not only been considered habit forming, but also addictive: in fact, although caffeine has occasionally been considered a drug of abuse, its potential for dependence has long been debated. At present, due to the scarcity of clinical evidence on caffeine dependence or abuse, no such diagnoses are included in the Substance Use Disorders section of the *Diagnostic and Statistical Manual of Mental Disorders IV* edition-TR (APA 2000). The recently published DSM-5 does not include caffeine use disorder, although research shows that as little as two to three cups of coffee can trigger a withdrawal effect marked by tiredness or sleepiness. There is sufficient evidence to support this as a condition; however, it is not yet clear to what extent it is a clinically significant disorder. To encourage further research on the impact of this condition, caffeine use disorder is included in Section III of DSM-5, among Conditions for Further Study—that is, proposed conditions that had clear merit but ultimately were judged to need further research before they might be considered as formal disorders. Inclusion of caffeine use disorder in Section III relates to the potential addictive behaviour caused by excessive, sustained consumption of caffeine and was contingent on the amount of empirical evidence available on a diagnosis, diagnostic reliability or validity, a clear clinical need, and potential benefit in advancing research (APA 2013).

Caffeine Misuse in Normal Populations

Actually, caffeine use is highly represented even in non-clinical samples, not surprisingly considering the widespread availability of caffeinated beverages, apparently in order to intensify vigilance and to increase attention. Energy drink consumption is common among college students, especially males, and has been associated with a variety of health-risk behaviours, and a greater body mass index (BMI) (Poulos and Pasch 2015). Excessive sugar-sweetened beverage (SSB) consumption has been associated with overweight and obesity. Caffeine is a common additive to SSB, and, through dependence effects, it has the potential to promote the consumption of caffeine-containing foods. In fact, the addition of low concentrations of caffeine to the SSB significantly increases the consumption of the SSB, and regulating caffeine as a food additive may be an effective strategy to decrease the consumption of nutrient-poor high-energy foods and beverages (Keast et al. 2015). Another study of college men and women examining the tendency for individuals to overlap addictions to common substances including caffeine and activities (i.e. exercise, gambling) found that self-esteem was positively related to exercise but unrelated to other addictions. Several gender differences in addictive tendencies were also revealed: men scored higher than women on addiction to alcohol, cigarettes, gambling, television, and Internet use, but women scored higher on caffeine and chocolate (Greenberg et al. 1999). Caffeine use is widespread in athletes as young as 11 years of age who are seeking athletic advantage over fellow competitors as it is inexpensive, readily available, medically quite safe, socially acceptable, and by most measures legal (Sinclair and Geiger 2000). Indeed, there is increasing concern about the potential adverse effects of caffeine on children: findings from the Kantar Worldpanel(KWP) Beverage Consumption Panel and the NHANES showed that caffeine consumption prevalence was generally consistent across studies and over time; more than one-half of 2- to 5-year-olds and ~75 % of older children (>5 years) consumed caffeine. The usual intakes of caffeine were 25 and 50 mg/d for children and adolescents aged 2–11 and 12–17 years, respectively (NHANES 2007–2010). Caffeine consumption is correlated with age and was higher in non-Hispanic white children. The key sources of caffeine were soda and tea as well as flavoured dairy (for children aged <12 years) and coffee (for those aged ≥12 years). The frequency of Caffeine Containing Energy Drinks (CCED)8383 use varied (2–30 %) depending on study setting, methods, and demographic characteristics. A statistically significant but small decline in caffeine intake was noted in children overall during the 10- to 12-year period examined; intakes remained stable among older children (≥12 years). A significant increasing trend in CCED and coffee consumption and a decline in soda intake were noted (1999–2010). In 2009–2010, 10 % of 12- to 19-year-olds and 10–25 % of caffeine consumers (aged 12–19 years) had intakes exceeding Canadian maximal guidelines (Ahluwalia and Herrick 2015).

Recently health warnings have been issued in a number of countries due to increasing reports of caffeine intoxication from energy drinks, and it seems likely that problems with caffeine dependence and withdrawal will also increase (Satel 2006; Ogawa and Ueki 2007; Reissig et al. 2009). Since 1999, in fact, several groups have analysed nutritional supplements with mass spectrometric methods (GC/MS, LC/MS/MS) for contaminations and adulterations with doping substances. These investigations showed that nutritional supplements contained prohibited stimulants such as ephedrines, caffeine, methylenedioxymethamphetamine, and sibutramine, which were not declared on the labels (Geyer et al. 2008). Intentional or unintentional caffeine abuse due to excessive intake of beverages or energy drinks containing caffeine is relatively frequent. Though death due to caffeine intoxication is rare, fatalities from caffeine toxicity—often due to the ingestion of caffeine tablets in the form of a weight-loss supplement—can occur (Mrvos et al. 1989; Takeuchi et al. 2007\; Bonsignore et al. 2014; Łukasik-Głebocka et al. 2012).

Caffeine and Psychiatric Disorders

Large amounts and long-term use of caffeine have been related to psychopathology (Lucas et al. 1990; Rihs et al. 1996; Ogawa and Ueki 2007; Ciapparelli et al. 2009) and it has been suggested that, in both normal and vulnerable subjects, caffeine can act as a trigger for psychiatric symptoms from anxiety to depression, and even psychosis (Broderick and Benjamin 2004). On the contrary, a reduction in caffeine intake seems to have a role in preventing psychiatric symptoms (Lambert et al. 2007 Caykoylu et al. 1997).

Excessive coffee consumption and its possible significance have long been discussed in relation to patients with psychiatric disorders including schizophrenia, affective disorders, sleep disorders, eating disorders, substance use disorders, as well as suicidal behaviours (Furlong 1975; Winstead 1976; Henderson et al. 2006; Boulenger et al. 1984; Greden et al. 1978; Sours 1983; Lucas et al. 1990; Baethge et al. 2009). Note that caffeine is metabolized by the hepatic cytochrome P-450 12 enzymes (CYP1A2), with an inhibitory effect on these enzymes; thus, negative effects may result from the interaction of caffeine with the kynetics of commonly prescribed psychotropic drugs—for instance, clozapine and molecules of some antidepressants (Carrillo and Benitez 2000).

Caffeine intake can be elevated to counteract sedation due to neuroleptic treatment in chronic psychotic patients or to facilitate mood changes in depression (Broderick et al. 2005). Ciapparelli et al. (2009) found similar caffeine intake among subjects suffering from different psychiatric disorders compared to healthy controls, but with a significantly higher maximum lifetime intake in the former. On the other hand, patients with anxiety disorders, especially those with panic-agoraphobic spectrum symptomatology, often show a tendency to caffeine avoidance due to an excessive sensibility to its stimulant effect that may trigger anxiety symptoms even at low dosages (Boulenger et al. 1984; Cassano et al. 1997).

Caffeine Use in Eating Disorders

Eating disorder (ED) patients often display excessive drinking, mainly non-alcoholic. The main reasons for consuming fluids were for fullness and appetite suppression; for feelings of control including feeling empty; to assist with purging; and for physiological reasons such as drinking when thirsty, after exercising and to increase energy levels via caffeine ingestion (Hart et al. 2011).

Among these patients, caffeine typically represents an energetic substitute without calories and a means to reduce hunger, lose weight, and increase vigilance. Caffeine does have some potentially beneficial physiologic effects, such as appetite suppression, increased metabolism, increased stimulant and diuretic action, increased muscle work output for endurance activities and delayed onset of fatigue. Caffeine intake, together with many other substances, may be observed both during starvation to guarantee "low-calorie" energy and in attempts to influence weight and appetite (Keys et al. 1950; Sours 1983; Faye and Treasure 1991; Krüger and Bräunig 1995).

Data from literature show an excess of heavy caffeine consumers or abusers among ED patients compared to individuals in the general population, but are controversial as regards the association with a specific subtype. Some studies have linked caffeine intake with purging subtypes and other dyscontrol behaviours such as alcohol or cigarette use (Charney et al. 1985; Krahn et al. 1991; Haug et al. 2001; Stock et al. 2002), while others found that caffeine consumption in young girls with ED differs from healthy ones only in presence of anorexia nervosa (Striegel-Moore et al. 2006).

The susceptibility of anorexic patients to caffeine abuse has also been described with an intoxication syndrome characterized by agitation, irritability, restlessness, confusion, rigidity, posturing, convulsions, coma, psychosis, hyperactivity, increased energy, muscle tension, anxiety, insomnia, abdominal pain, and vomiting resulting from the pharmacologic actions of high doses of caffeine, which is exacerbated in low-weight subjects (Sours 1983; Shaul et al. 1984). Restricting the purging behaviours of anorexic patients who have developed them served to increase their caffeine intake, presumably as an expression of their experience of losing control rather than as a form of food-antidote. In contrast, caffeine use in Binge Eating Disorder (BED) patients does not represent an attempt to self-medicate to suppress appetite, as it does in AN and Bulima Nervosa (BN) patients, just as BED patients do not use other mechanisms of compensation and neutralization. Instead, caffeine assumption in these patients seems more related to their passive attitude towards overeating, although highly dissatisfied with their body appearance (Burgalassi et al. 2009).

A high percentage of ED patients ordinarily use caffeine with an average intake similar to that of the general population, but they are more prone to binging. In fact, when considering caffeine abuse and average intake during periods of heavy consumption, ED patients showed a significantly higher prevalence than healthy controls, with an excess especially among purging subtypes. Furthermore, caffeine intake was probably related to the psychopathological dimension of dyscontrol rather than to the severity of the ED. Among heavy drinkers, a positive association between daily caffeine intake and alcohol and cigarette use is also reported, suggesting a link with the dimension of impulse dysregulation. As regards comorbidity, data from the literature suggest a causal relationship between higher caffeine intake for self-medication and comorbid anxiety and depression; and a higher use of caffeine as self-medication a positive correlation with caffeine intake; note that when started on therapy, some patients (20 %) showed a decrease in caffeine intake (Charney et al. 1985; Krahn et al. 1991; Haug et al. 2001; Burgalassi et al. 2009).

Other studies examined caffeine use and caffeine dependence and risk for the symptoms, or diagnosis, of psychiatric disorders. Bergin and Kendler (2012) specifically investigated shared common genetic or environmental factors with caffeine use, caffeine tolerance, or caffeine withdrawal and Generalized Anxiety Disorder (GAD), panic disorder, phobias, Major Depressive Disorder (MDD) and AN or BN. In their model the genetic correlation between AN, BN, and caffeine tolerance were 0.64 and 0.49, respectively. However, removal of the genetic and environmental correlation parameters resulted in significantly worse-fitting models for GAD, phobias, MDD, AN, and BN, demonstrating that there was suggestive evidence of shared genetic and environmental liability between psychiatric disorders and caffeine phenotypes.

The psychopathological dimension of addiction has long been investigated in ED. Research shows a significant association between ED and substance use disorders (SUD). Substances other than caffeine, such as tobacco, insulin, thyroid medications, stimulants or over-the-counter medications (laxatives, diuretics), may be used to aid weight loss and/or provide energy, and alcohol or psychoactive substances are used for emotional regulation or as part of a pattern of impulsive behavior. ED patients who abuse substances demonstrate worse ED symptomatology and poorer outcomes than those with EDs alone, including increased general medical complications and psychopathology, longer recovery times, poorer functional outcomes, and higher relapse rates. Furthermore, results suggest an important difference in the chronology of EDs and SUDs: women with BN may be turning to substances to dampen bulimic urges, whereas those with AN may be engaging in substance use initially in an effort to lose weight. Results also suggest that familial factors contribute to the comorbidity between BN and SUD (Baker et al. 2010). A key message conveyed in the current literature is the importance of screening and assessment for comorbid SUDs and addictive behaviours comprehensive of caffeine, thyroid medications, diuretics, and laxatives in patients presenting with either ED, for possible therapeutic implications. Overall, the literature indicates that the ED and SUD should be addressed simultaneously using a multi-disciplinary approach (Gregorowski et al. 2013).

Conclusions

Research studies do not directly investigate the relationship between caffeine use or misuse and issues concerning body appearance or perceived body image, though there is rich data concerning weight loss both in clinical and normal populations. In any case, a link can be found when considering the dimension of self-esteem. Caffeine, in fact, is a psychoactive substance that is inexpensive, legal, and morally accepted and helps in increasing energy, reactiveness, and endurance and indirectly sustaining a sense of self-efficacy. At the same time, caffeine suppresses the appetite and helps in weight control, especially in individuals on the anorexic-bulimic spectrum, even those who do not have a full-blown eating disorder. Thus, through its wide-ranging physiological and psychological effects, caffeine can help in sustaining self-esteem in social contexts that emphasize appearance, competition, and performance, but users are nevertheless burdened with a self-reinforcement effect and a potential risk of addiction.

References

Ahluwalia, N., & Herrick, K. (2015). Caffeine intake from food and beverage sources and trends among children and adolescents in the United States: Review of national quantitative studies from 1999 to 2011. *Advances in Nutrition: An International Review Journal, 6*(1): 102–1111.

American Psychiatric Association. (2000). *Diagnostic and statistical manual of mental disorders* (4th ed.). Washington, DC: American Psychiatric Publising.

American Psychiatric Association. (2013). *Diagnostic and statistical manual of mental disorders* (5th ed.). Arlington, VA: American Psychiatric Publishing.

Baker, J. H., Mitchell, K. S., Neale, M. C., & Kendler, K. S. (2010). Eating disorder symptomatology and substance use disorders: Prevalence and shared risk in a population based twin sample. *International Journal of Eating Disorders, 43*(7), 648–658.

Baethge, C., Tondo, L., Lepri, B., & Baldessarini, R. J. (2009). Coffee and cigarette use: association with suicidal acts in 352 Sardinian bipolar disorder patients. *Bipolar Disord, 1*(5), 494–503.

Bergin, J. E., & Kendler, K. S. (2012). Common psychiatric disorders and caffeine use, tolerance, and withdrawal: An examination of shared genetic and environmental effects. *Twin Research and Human Genetics, 5*(4), 473–482.

Bolton, S., & Null, G. (1981). Caffeine: Psychological effects, use and abuse. *Orthomolecular Psychiatry, 10*(3), 202–211.

Bonsignore, A., Sblano, S., Pozzi, F., Ventura, F., Dell'Erba, A., & Palmiere, C. (2014). A case of suicide by ingestion of caffeine. *Forensic Science Medicine and Pathology, 10*(3), 448–451.

Boulenger, J. P., Uhde, T. W., Wolff, E. A., & R.M., P. (1984). Increased sensitivity to caffeine in patients with panic disorders; Preliminary evidence. *Archives of General Psychiatry, 41*, 1067–1071.

Broderick, P. J., & Benjamin, A. B. (2004). Caffeine and psychiatric symptoms: A review. *The Journal of the Oklahoma State Medical Association, 97*, 538–542.

Broderick, P. J., Benjamin, A. B., & Dennis, L. W. (2005). Caffeine and psychiatric medication interactions: A review. *The Journal of the Oklahoma State Medical Association, 98*(8), 380–384.

Burgalassi, A. Ramacciotti, C. E., Bianchi, M., Coli, E., Polese, L., Bondi, E., Massimetti, G., Dell'osso, L. (2009). Caffeine consumption among eating disorder patients: Epidemiology, motivations, and potential of abuse *Eating and Weight Disorders-Studies on Anorexia, Bulimia and Obesity, 14*(4): e212–e21e218.

Carrillo, J. A., & Benitez, J. (2000). Clinically significant pharmacokinetic interactions between dietary caffeine and medications. *Clinical Pharmacokinetics, 39*(2), 127–153.

Cassano, G. B., Michelini, S., Shear, M. K., Coli, E., Maser, J. D., & Frank, E. (1997). The panic-agorophobic spectrum: A descriptive approach to the assessment and treatment of subtle symptoms. *American Journal of Psychiatry, 154*(5), 27–38.

Caykoylu, A., Ekinci, O., & Kuloglu, M. (1997). Improvement from treatment-resistant schizoaffective disorder, manic type after stopping heavy caffeine intake: A case report. *Progress in Neuro-Psychopharmacology and Biological Psychiatry, 32*, 1349–1350.

Charney, D. S., Heninger, G. R., & Jatlow, P. I. (1985). Increased anxiogenic effects of caffeine in panic disorders. *Archives of General Psychiatry, 42*, 233–243.

Ciapparelli, A., Paggini, R., Carmassi, C., Taponecco, C., Consoli, G., Ciampa, G., et al. (2009). Patterns of caffeine consumption in psychiatric patients. An Italian study. *European Psychiatry, 25*(4), 230–235.
Faye, T. A., & Treasure, J. (1991). Caffeine abuse in bulimia nervosa. *International Journal of Eating Disorders, 10*, 373–377.
Fredholm, B. B. (1998). Adenosine, adenosine receptors and the actions of caffeine. *Pharmacology & Toxicology, 76*(2), 93–101.
Furlong, F. W. (1975). Possible psychiatric significance of excessive coffee consumption. *The Canadian Psychiatric Association Journal/La Revue de l'Association des psychiatres du Canada, 20*(8), 577–583.
Geyer, H., Parr, M. K., Koehler, K., Marek, U., Schänzer, W., & Thevis, M. (2008). Nutritional supplements cross-contaminated and faked with doping substances. *Journal of Mass Spectrometry, 43*(7), 892–902.
Graham, T. E. (2001). Caffeine and exercise: Metabolism, endurance and performance. *Sports Medicine, 31*, 785–807.
Graham, T. E., Sathasivam, P., Rowland, M., Marko, N., Greer, F., & Battram, D. (2001). Caffeine ingestion elevates plasma insulin response in humans during anoral glucose tolerance test. *Canadian Journal of Physiology and Pharmacology, 79*(1), 559–565.
Greden, J. F., Fontaine, P., Lubetsky, M., & Chamberlin, K. (1978). Anxiety and depression associated with caffeinism among psychiatric inpatients. *American Journal of Psychiatry, 135*, 963–966.
Greenberg, J. L., Lewis, S. E., & Dodd, D. K. (1999). Overlapping addictions and self-esteem among college men and women. *Addictive Behaviours, 24*(4), 565–571.
Greer, F., Hudson, R., Ross, R., & Graham, T. E. (2001). Caffeine ingestion decreases glucose disposal during a hyperinsulinemic-euglycemic clamp in sedentary humans. *Diabetes, 50*, 2349–2354.
Gregorowski, C., Seedat, S., & Jordaan, G. P. (2013). A clinical approach to the assessment and management of co-morbid eating disorders and substance use disorders. *BMC Psychiatry., 7*(13), 289.
Griffiths, R. R., & Woodson, P. P. (1988). Reinforcing properties of caffeine: Studies in humans and laboratory animals. *Pharmacology Biochemistry and Behavior, 29*(2), 419–427.
Han, D. H., Hansen, P. A., Nolte, L. A., & Holloszy, J. O. (1998). Removal of adenosine decreases the responsiveness of muscle glucose transport to insulin and contractions. *Diabetes, 47*, 1671–1675.
Hart, S., Abraham, S., Franklin, R. C., & Russell, J. (2011). The reasons why eating disorder patients drink. *European Eating Disorders Review, 19*(2), 121–128.

Haug, N. A., Heiberg, L. J., & Guarda, A. S. (2001). Cigarette smoking and substance use among eating disordered inpatients. *Eating and Weight Disorders-Studies on Anorexia, Bulimia and Obesity, 6*(3), 130–139.

Henderson, D. C., Borba, C. P., Daley, T. B., Boxill, R., Nguyen, D. D., Culhane, M. A., et al. (2006). Dietary intake profile of patients with schizophrenia. *Annals of Clinical Psychiatry, 18*(2), 99–105.

Hughes, J. R., Oliveto, A. H., Liguori, A., Carpenter, J., & Howard, T. (1998). Endorsement of DSM-IV dependence criteria among caffeine users. *Drug and Alcohol Dependence, 52*(2), 99–107.

Keast, R. S., Swinburn, B. A., Sayompark, D., Whitelock, S., & Riddell, L. J. (2015). Caffeine increases sugar-sweetened beverage consumption in a free-living population: A randomised controlled trial. *British Journal of Nutrition, 113*(2), 366–371.

Keijzers, G. B., Galan, B. E. D., Tack, C. J., & Smits, P. (2002). Caffeine can decrease insulin sensitivity in humans. *Diabetes Care, 25*, 364–369.

Keys, A., Brožek, J., Henschel, A., Mickelsen, O., & Taylor, H. L. (1950). *The biology of human starvation*. Minneapolis: University of Minnesota Press.

Krahn, D. D., Hasse, S., Ray, A., Gosnell, B., & Drewnowski, A. (1991). Caffeine consumption in patients with eating disorders. *Psychiatric Services, 42*(3), 313–315.

Krüger, S., & Bräunig, P. (1995). Abuse of body weight reducing agents in bulimia nervosa. *Der Nervenarzt, 66*(1), 66–69.

Lambert, Ra., Harvey, I., & Poland, F. (2007). A pragmatic, unblinded randomised controlled trial comparing an occupational therapy-led lifestyle approach and routine GP care for panic disorder treatment in family care. *Journal of Affective Disorders, 99*(1–3), 63–71.

Lucas, P. B., Pickar, D., Kelsoe, J., Rapaport, M., Pato, C., & Hommer, D. (1990). Effects of the acute administration of caffeine in patients with schizophrenia. *Biological Psychiatry, 28*(1), 35–40.

Łukasik-Głebocka, M., Sommerfeld, K., Tezyk, A., & Zielińska-Psuja, B. (2012). Acute poisoning with weight-loss dietary supplement falsely suggesting the use of amphetamine. *Przegląd lekarski, 70*(10), 880–883.

Mrvos, R. M., Reilly, P. E., Dean, B. S., & Krenzelok, E. P. (1989). Massive caffeine ingestion resulting in death. *Veterinary and Human Toxicology, 31*(6), 571–572.

Ogawa, N., & Ueki, H. (2007). Clinical importance of caffeine dependence and abuse. *Psychiatry and Clinical Neurosciences, 61*(3), 263–268.

Petrie, H. J., Chown, S. E., Belfie, L. M., Duncan, A. M., McLaren, D. H., Conquer, J. A., et al. (2004). Caffeine ingestion increases the insulin response to an oral-glucose-tolerance test in obese men before and after weight loss. *The American Journal of Clinical Nutrition, 80*(1), 22–28.

Poulos, N. S., & Pasch, K. E. (2015). Energy drink consumption is associated with unhealthy dietary behaviours among college youth. *Perspectives in Public Health*.

Reissig, C. J., Strain, E. C., & Griffiths, R. R. (2009). Caffeinated energy drinks—A growing problem. *Drug and Alcohol Dependence, 99*(1), 1–10.

Rihs, M., Müller, C., & Baumann, P. (1996). Caffeine consumption in hospitalized psychiatric patients. *European archives of Psychiatry and Clinical Neuroscience, 246*(2), 83–92.

Satel, S. (2006). Is caffeine addictive?—A review of the literature. *The American Journal of Drug and Alcohol Abuse, 32*(4), 493–502.

Shaul, P. W., Farrell, M. K., & Maloney, M. J. (1984). Caffeine toxicity as a cause of acute psychosis in anorexia nervosa. *The Journal of Pediatrics, 105*(3), 493–495.

Sinclair, C. J. D., & Geiger, J. D. (2000). Caffeine use in sports: A pharmacological review. *Journal of Sports Medicine and Physical Fitness, 40*(1), 71.

Sours, J. A. (1983). Case reports of anorexia nervosa and caffeinism. *American Journal of Psychiatry, 140*, 235–236.

Stock, S. L., Goldberg, E., Corbett, S., & Katzman, D. K. (2002). Substance use in female adolescents with eating disorders. *Journal of Adolescent Health, 31*(2), 176–182.

Strain, E. C., Mumford, G. K., Silverman, K., & Griffiths, R. R. (1994). Caffeine dependence syndrome: Evidence from case histories and experimental evaluations. *Jama, 272*(13), 1043–1048.

Striegel-Moore, R. H., Franko, D. L., Thompson, D., Barton, B., Schreiber, G. B., & Daniels, S. R. (2006). Caffeine intake in eating disorders. *International Journal of Eating Disorders, 39*(2), 162–165.

Takeuchi, S., Homma, M., Inoue, J., Kato, H., Murata, K., & Ogasawara, T. (2007). Case of intractable ventricula fibrillation by a multicomponent dietary supplement containing ephedra and caffeine overdose. *Chudoku kenkyu: Chudoku Kenkyukai jun kikanshi = The Japanese Journal of Toxicology, 20*(3), 269–271.

Thong, F. S., & Graham, T. E. (2002a). Caffeine-induced impairment of glucose tolerance is abolished by β-adrenergic receptor blockade in humans. *Journal of Applied Physiology, 92*(6), 2347–2352.

Thong, F. S., & Graham, T. E. (2002b). The putative roles of adenosine in insulin-and exercise-mediated regulation of glucose transport and glycogen metabolism in skeletal muscle. *Canadian Journal of Applied Physiology, 27*(2), 152–178.

Thong, F. S., Derave, W., Kiens, B., Graham, T. E., Ursø, B., Wojtaszewski, J. F., et al. (2002). Caffeine-induced impairment of insulin action but not insulin signaling in human skeletal muscle is reduced by exercise. *Diabetes, 51*(3), 583–590.

Vergauwen, L., Hespel, P., & Richter, E. A. (1994). Adenosine receptors mediate synergistic stimulation of glucose uptake and transport by insulin and by contractions in rat skeletal muscle. *Journal of Clinical Investigation, 93*(3), 974.

Winstead, D. K. (1976). Coffee consumption among psychiatric inpatients. *The American Journal of Psychiatry, 133*(12), 1447–1450.

6

Body Image, Enhancement, and Health in the Advertising of Sports and Nutritional Supplements

Simon Outram

Enhance Your Every Day: Rely on [XX] as a potent everyday multi-vitamin to help keep you on your A-game.

Increased ATP production for maximum energy output. Improved anaerobic and aerobic performance for speed, power and endurance.

With my busy schedule, it's important to keep my immune system strong so I take a premium quality probiotic to keep my digestive system healthy and give my immune system a boost.

Complete Multi-Vitamin. Helps you cope with stress and boosts your immune system. Rich in antioxidants. Boosts energy levels.

(Advertisements for Supplements found in *Men's Health* Magazine, 2012–2013)

S. Outram (✉)
817B Edwards Street, Chapel Hill, NC 27516, USA

© The Editor(s) (if applicable) and The Author(s) 2016
M. Hall et al. (eds.), *Chemically Modified Bodies*,
DOI 10.1057/978-1-137-53535-1_6

Introduction

A walk through any retail supermarket or pharmacy will attest to the size of the market for nutritional and sports supplements, including sports drinks. Data backs up the perception that the market for sports and nutritional supplements is both substantial and has been growing. Approximately 40–60% of the US population use supplements, with the use of supplements growing rapidly in many other Western nations over the past 20 to 30 years (Bailey et al. 2011; Dascombe et al. 2010; Dickinson et al. 2014; Gahche et al. 2011; Garcia-Alvarez et al. 2014; Reinert et al. 2007; Ritchie 2007). Advertising through body image plays a key part in the appeal of such products. Images of physically fit young men and women dominate the sports supplements and sports drinks sector of the market while images of both young and old enjoying healthy activities regularly feature in the advertising of vitamins and other health-maintaining or augmenting nutritional supplements. In the following chapter, the author uses examples of supplement advertising found in the popular health and lifestyle magazine *Men's Health* to focus upon how image—particularly that of young and physically active men—provides both an incentive for the consumption of such products and reflects an appeal to a particular type of health-related behaviour concerned with physical and mental enhancement.

Body Image, Body Dissatisfaction, and Advertising

Prior to engaging more fully with the issues arising from supplement use as a form of enhancement, it is worth highlighting the connection between supplement advertising and body image and the significance of this connection for health; a health-enhancement theme that we will return to throughout this chapter.

Men's Health magazine is dominated by body image. Photos of tall and strong young men are found across a majority of the covers of the magazine and the inner pages (along with stereotypically smaller and attractive women). Not surprisingly, body imagery also plays a key role in the content of the advertising contained within the magazine, including advertising for sports and nutritional supplements. Of the approximately 100 supplement advertisements reviewed for this chapter (found in the 24 monthly issues of *Men's Health* Magazine; 2012–2013 Australian Edition) 60 featured men being physically active. Particularly frequently used images included men lifting weights, running or training for sport, or posed photos of men with extremely well-defined upper bodies. Images of strong and athletic sports and/or TV personalities are also featured in multiple advertisements. (The other dominant advertisement image was of the product itself—the bottle or container as likely to be seen on store shelves).

Significant concerns have been raised with respect to the health impact of such images on individual readers (Botta 2003; Hatoum and Belle 2004; Field et al. 2005; Hargreaves and Tiggemann 2004; Morry and Staska 2001). It has been argued by several observers that repeated exposure to such imagery *may* be deleterious to mental (and physical) health. As Blond (2008) has argued, existing research "suggest[s] that men who are dissatisfied with their appearance are at increased risk for image induced body dissatisfaction" even if "men who are satisfied with their appearance may be protected against this exposure to images". Similarly, Agliata and Tantleff-Dunn (2004) have argued that while "little empirical evidence exists regarding media's direct impact on males' body image, research does suggest that the rate of body image dissatisfaction among males may be increasing".

Above and beyond the direct impact of such images on readers, it has been argued that a growing number of young men generally may be impacted by the body image norms created by such magazines. Research conducted by Labre (2005) suggests that "both readers and non-readers of fitness magazines described the societal ideal as lean and moderately muscular". The parallels with female body image found in magazines are self-evident with the stereotypical images of women found within such magazines conditioning what is considered to be a desirable size and shape for women more generally (Cusumano and Thompson 1997; Tiggemann and McGill 2004). Linking this gendered physical stereotyping with the rise of *Men's Health* and associated male health and lifestyle magazines, Dworkin and Wachs (2009) refer to a widespread societal concern or obsession over bodily imperfection and specifically to a magazine culture for men whereby they are encouraged to "confess their gendered failures". In short, the growth in the market for such magazines both reflects and re-enforces a notion that there is a crisis in male health which needs to be overcome (Crawshaw 2007; Gough 2006; Stibbe 2004). Magazines such as *Men's Health* offer a variety of products through which such failures—the failure to be as big, strong, and handsome as these ideal male stereotypes—can at least partially be overcome. Thus, Alexander (2003) has argued that a whole "male body" industry sector has emerged "that seek[s] profits built on male insecurities".

By way of summary, there is little doubt that dietary and nutritional supplement advertisers (among others) are keen to nurture and commercially exploit male insecurity about body size and shape. While many of those reading such magazines may already be keen to adopt the types of training regime that will ultimately provide them with at least some measure of success in achieving their physical ideals, a great deal more (non-readers of such magazines) may be impacted upon by the images and idealized messages of such advertising and may feel pressure to conform to this stereotypical body standard.

Advertising, Enhancement, and Emerging Questions

As has been seen earlier, supplement advertising regularly features photos of men with bodies that that are well above the norm—enhanced—in terms of strength, agility, and stereotypical attractiveness. However, enhancement does not just feature within the images presented in such advertising. The accompanying text to the sports and nutritional supplement advertising reviewed includes multiple references to the terms associated with enhancing the body and/or the mind. Claims are made with respect to products that "enhance mental and physical performance", "enhance muscle tissue repair", and more generally to the ability to "enhance your day". Associated terms such as "boost", "improve", and "increase" all feature in advertising. It is argued, therefore, that questions pertaining to enhancement—questions that emerge both in the physical and mental contexts of enhancement—can and should be applied to supplement advertising and supplement use.

Bostrom and Sandberg (2009), argue that "most efforts to enhance cognition are of a rather mundane nature, and some have been practised for thousands of years. The prime example is education and training where the goal is often not only to impart specific skills or information, but also to improve general mental faculties such as concentration, memory, and critical thinking". As for internal forms of enhancement, they refer to caffeine as "herbal extracts reputed to improve memory" and "energy drinks" as forms of commonly found enhancement products "all vying for consumers who are hoping to turbo-charge their brains". Within capitalist economics we might view enhancement as closely related to consumer choice. By way of illustration, people constantly try to 'enhance' their quality of life by various purchases—a second car, a bigger TV. The advertising and use of supplements may—at one level— be seen as fitting this generalizable and somewhat 'mundane' pattern of enhancement.

More controversially, enhancement has come to be discussed as an issue of performance enhancement drug use in sport (Hemphill 2009; Outram 2013; Petróczi and Aidman 2008) and cognitive enhancement—the use of medications by persons without prescription for the purposes of augmenting mental capacities (Cakic 2009; Greely et al. 2008; McCabe et al. 2005). With respect to the former (sports) context, particular attention has been paid to so-called doping and the regulation of performance-enhancing drugs which separates out licit performance-enhancing drug use from illicit supplement use. Within sport, the prohibition of by the World Anti-Doping Agency is based upon the criteria of achieving performance benefits, being detrimental to health, and contradicting what is referred to as "the spirit of sport" (WADA 2015). Mirroring the rationale for drug prohibition in sport some bioethicists have questioned whether students should be tested for the use of such cognitively enhancing substances when taking exams, in part based upon whether the results of the tests might be seen as 'inauthentic' or forms of cheating (Cakic 2009; Parens 2005; Schermer 2008). Supplement advertising and use can also, therefore, be seen as part of this more controversial arena within which the limits of enhancement are discussed in terms of regulation and the ethical acceptability of use.

In summary it is argued that by applying the concept of enhancement to supplement advertising and the use of supplements it is possible to link concerns over the health impact of body image to readers and non-readers of such magazines to questions concerned with what it means to enhance physical and mental prowess through the use of substances within sport and, in a related manner within society. Moreover, questions can be asked regarding the consequences of such enhancement on the health of individuals and perceptions of health within society. Within the specific context of sport, supplement use may be questioned as to whether it is a form of cheating within sport (this is a question for sports ethicists and regulators—some of whom have already challenged the ethical and practical issues associated with anti-doping regulation—see Hemphill 2009; Kayser et al. 2007; Smith and Stewart 2008). As has been seen earlier, questions concerned with cognitive enhancement and cheating may also apply to academic testing. More widely, the use of supplements prompts questions as to whether it is fair for some persons to have access to products that may enhance their health but others are excluded from these benefits on the basis of cost? Conversely, it might be asked whether there is potential for persons to be coerced into using cognitively and/or physically enhancing substances of this type (see Forlini and Racine 2009; Simon 1984 for discussion of coercion in both contexts). Thus analysing supplement advertising as a form of enhancement-advertising opens up a range of ethical questions concerned with regulation, social impact, and health; noting that body image provides the key platform by which supplement advertisers appeal to this sense of enhancement objective.

The Merging of Enhancement with Health

Questions are already being asked within the medical profession as to whether physicians should be providing medications specifically for the purposes of enhancement (Banjo et al. 2010; Hotze et al. 2011; Larriviere et al. 2009). As previously discussed, similar questions may be asked of supplements (should they be supplied to all?) given their close association with enhancement (arguably such questions should be foregrounded with questions pertaining to the realizable health benefits of using supplements—see Bent 2008; Marik and Flemmer 2012 for discussion of the efficacy of supplements). Underlying these questions are concerns over whether the legitimation of some forms of novel enhancement (perhaps including the growing use of supplements) are transforming what might be seen as legitimate or necessary forms of treatment (see Morgan 2009; Wolpe 2002). Put another way, to what extent does the normalization of using certain products to enhance our physical and mental wellbeing become less of an option and more of a social or even medical necessity?

Excerpts from the nutritional supplement advertisements featured in *Men's Health* highlight the integral nature of the health claims made alongside the imagery and text of enhancement. Some health-enhancement claims are quasi-therapeutic such as supplement advertising that suggest the product can be used to "promote complete hydration", "promote strong bone and teeth", or "promote natural restful sleep". Others rely on slightly less specific claims regarding boosting or maintaining the "immune function" and appeals to physical and mental health such as product claims for "general wellbeing and vitality" and "help[ing] enhance mental and physical performance". It is also worth highlighting how all four of the advertisements featured at the start of this chapter combine elements of enhancement along with generalized health claims—boosting, maximizing, and enhancing along with generalized health claims. Other examples of this combined appeal to enhancement and health include the following, "Whether you're an athlete or working out around a hectic lifestyle, [XX] can help keep you fuelled and performing at your best". Another product claims that it "replenishes natural stores in your body that can be depleted by stress or an intense training regime" and "helps support your capacity to cope with stress and maintain your general health and wellbeing".

Two directly related issues that have arisen in the context of supplement advertising. The first concerns the wording of such health-associated claims and the second explores the perception of supplement users regarding the health benefits of supplements. Briefly described, only structural-functional claims can be made for the use of supplements unless specific evidence of therapeutic efficacy is provided (akin to pharmaceutical regulation). Thus terms such as "helping", "promoting", and "assisting" are frequently seen in association with supplement use, rather than direct claims to alleviating symptoms. The wording of claims continues to be the subject of considerable debate (DeLorme et al. 2012; Mason and Scammon 2000). Perhaps more significantly, a number of studies have been undertaken which suggest that despite restrictions on the language used to promote and label supplements, many people are apt to simply assume that supplements are de-facto treatments for mild conditions such as irregular sleeplessness and anxiety (Mason and Scammon 2011; Rotfeld 2009). Indeed, notwithstanding the regulatory role played in separating pharmaceutical claims from the structural-functional claims allowable for nutritional supplement advertisement, Thompson and Nichter (2007) have found that "consumers can decode the specific ambiguity of the structure and function claims to locate a potential treatment for almost any health condition". In effect, enhancement *and* health concepts are merged in such advertising. In the following paragraphs a variety of concerns over the merging of enhancement with health are discussed.

Miah (2007) has described how health in the context of elite sport is a distinct variant on how the general population might consider to be a healthy state; athletes (and sport-physicians) are first and foremost concerned with achieving health for a specific purpose not for their longer term wellbeing. While one may be comfortable that elite sportspersons suffer some forms of health damage (repeated injuries) in pursuit of their goals as they are well paid and do so willingly, it is considerably more disconcerting to think that the average person may be subscribing to a similar form of short-term health objective. Concerns over what might be called sports-orientated or enhancement-specific health reflect the problematic relationship between sport, health, and exercise. In short, the maximization of physical potential in the elite sports context does not necessarily equate to good health (Murphy and Waddington 1998; Waddington et al. 1997). This is not to say that sport is unhealthy or that the ethos of sport and sports performance should be singled out as especially socially damaging, but instead to re-iterate that health and sport are not synonymous. In a similar manner the maximization of mental output has come under scrutiny in discussions of cognitive enhancements with respect to mental health and social wellbeing. Discussants have questioned whether a cognitively enhanced society would necessarily be a 'healthier' society (kinder, more considerate, or fairer?) (Parens 1998; Persson and Savulescu 2008). In a more specific manner supplements, Lucke and Partridge (2013) have argued that cognitive enhancement—through stimulants—may offer the promise of minimizing the problems associated with daily cycles of tiredness and stress but do little to address the underlying health issues associated with chronic stress or lack of sleep. Evidently, "Executive Stress Formula", the name of one product advertised in *Men's Health* magazine, suggests the readers can cope with excessively long hours if they take this type of supplement (or at least may cope better) offers a similar promise.

An associated argument emerges with respect to how such advertising not only appeals to a particular sense of over-exertion (physical and mental) and health, but also that it may increase the likelihood of unhealthy or risky behaviour. Thus, while supplement advertising cannot be blamed for not solving the social issues of over-work and stress in the early twenty-first century, it can be questioned on the basis of how such advertising suggests that unhealthy lifestyle choices can be overcome using supplements. In Bolton et al.'s (2006) experimental study of healthy messaging and behaviours it was suggested that "various remedies (diet crazes, supplements, fat fighting drugs, and even surgery)" play a role in suggesting in the minds of users that that they can engage in risky behaviours (unhealthy behaviours) with only minimal consequences. As Bolton et al. (2006) state, "Put simply, remedy messages suggest that a 'get out of jail free card' is available to take the risk out of risky behaviour. Consumers trade away protective gain provided by the remedy through intentions to engage in more risky behaviour". In an analogous manner, sports and dietary supplement advertising encourages physical or mental over-exertion and then offers a remedy. This is particularly the case with respect to large number of advertisements featuring products that both boost energy and contain products that claim to aid physical recovery. A more direct version of this appeal to engage in over-exertion and potentially risky behaviour while balancing this out with a health-promoting supplement is found in an advertisement carried for a liver detoxifier.

The advertisement states somewhat benignly that it "contains premium quality herbs to support liver and aid detoxification" but is headlined by the personal 'advice' of a well-known sports personality that "at the end of a great night, spare a thought for tomorrow". The message is that you can drink alcohol to excess but not suffer the consequences. In a similar manner Nichter and Thompson's (2006) research into supplement users motivations for taking supplements found that "many of the young supplement users we talked with said that they took dietary supplements, especially vitamins, to counterbalance unhealthy lifestyle choices".

Supplements Advertising as a Mirror to Twenty-First Century Health

Bunton (1997) writes of "class of consumer" that has emerged within Western countries who is concerned about "healthy diets, staying in shape and *increasing body potential* [italics added]". Specifically referring to the role of supplements in this self-motivated physical self, Rose (2001) has referred to how the use of *"vitamins and dietary supplements* and the whole range of complementary, alternative and 'self-health' practices" [italics added] have emerged in this culture of autonomous healthcare while Bolton et al. (2008) have argued that "supplements may be seen as part of a broader array of complementary behaviours that must be engaged in to protect one's health".

While the promotion of self-health through supplement use and through other activities (the use of gyms, jogging, etc.) can largely be seen as positives in the fight against ill-health, concerns have been raised with respect to how the positive health movement has merged with what might be called an obligation for to take care of one's health to a level hitherto considered beyond the norm. As Rose (2001) argues during the late twentieth century in many advanced industrial societies "the very idea of health was re-figured—the will to health would not merely seek the avoidance of sickness or premature death, but would encode an optimization of one's corporeality to embrace a kind of overall 'well-being'". Thus, not only are we responsible for our personal health, we are conditioned to "optimize" our wellbeing—an optimisation which ties in with advertising that promotes the use of enhancing products. The integral part played by supplements with respect to taking responsibility for one's own health has been referred to by Nichter and Thompson (2006) with reference to how "even the 'token gesture' of taking supplements in the face of an adverse environment has come to signify a moral commitment to one's own health (Nichter 2003)". The choice to become healthy in an enhanced manner becomes less of a choice and more of a responsibility; with advertising in *Men's Health* reinforcing a message of active health promotion through purchasing a variety of health enhancement products including nutritional supplements.

In the final part of this chapter, the question that is posed is whether supplement advertising can be seen as mirroring and/or transforming concepts of health. Put another way, what does supplement advertising suggest about contemporary concepts of health among this population group (and perhaps more widely)? Three trends or health-concepts are discussed with respect to supplements advertising and what it might illuminate with respect to the direction of twenty-first century health in advanced capitalist societies; societies which are largely nutrient sufficient and relatively wealthy by global standards.

The first trend that might be seen is that of an *individualized* or personalized conceptualization of health. Pomeranz et al. (2014) has argued a key feature of nutritional supplement advertisements is the ability to present a picture of "flexible specificity" meaning that "even multivitamins must be tailored to fit an individual's specific needs". This review suggests that such flexible specificity can be found in references to the "highest grade" "high strength" which appeals to a sense of the product being special, thus making the person special. While it would be wrong to suggest that this appeal to the individual is somehow unique to supplement advertising, it does support the perception that the supplement market is largely based upon an individualized appeal to a sense of health (self-health rather than public health). Taking supplements does not make you unique (far from it), but taking them does indicate that the individual is prepared to find a product that suits them, or at least is advertised as fitting the individual's health requirements and objectives.

The second trend might be characterized as one in which health is *instantly accessible*. Quinones et al. (2013) have argued that the appeal of supplements to the US market is located in the desires of individuals "to lose weight, live longer, boost energy, prevent disease, think more clearly, be happier, sleep better, and build muscle-mass without taking the substantial time or effort or discipline that would be necessary to do so naturally". As Quinones et al. go on to say, "Keenly aware of this collective impatience, profit-driven supplement manufacturers entice consumers with promises of easy and rapid solutions". This review of supplement advertising suggests that sports and nutritional supplement purchases offer a commercial outlet whereby such objectives can be met in various forms—boosting or maintaining the immune system, enhancing muscle growth, maintaining energy throughout the day, and overcoming poor health decisions. Given that this review and analysis was conducted through advertising found in the Australian version of *Men's Health* it is suggested that these traits are not exclusive to US citizens.

Another way of phrasing this collective impatience regarding health achievement is that health has become a commodified entity (Henderson and Petersen 2002). Closely aligned to the sense of an individualized and tailored appeal to health, Nichter and Thompson (2006) have written that the US public is constantly exposed to products that send the messages "good health may be purchased at a cost" and "here is an easy way to take care of yourself". In short, the third trend which might be identified is that health is not only purchasable but that *not everyone can have access to the best health*. Supplement advertising is full of references to supplements that are of "premium quality" contain "premium" complex formulas, or provide a "unique combination" of vitamins. Such advertising encourages a sense the individual purchaser is being tailored to and, moreover, that not everyone is getting as good a product. There are multiple manners by which we might wish to analyse the benefits and problems associated with commodified health. We might applaud the fact that those with enough money are interested in looking after themselves; the active and healthy citizenship role (see above). We might also be somewhat neutral in accepting that there is nothing new in health inequities within nations and between nations. However, perhaps what is most concerning is that while supplement advertising is intimately connected to an appeal for healthiness, it is equally tied to a sense that this form of healthiness is *not* for all. Again turning to Nichter and Thompson's interview-based study of supplement use it is suggested that "despite comments and misgivings about health inequities being related to economic maldistribution, these supplement users expressed the idea that health consumerism cannot help but lead to good health" and how "those with more money are probably going to live longer than those with less in today's world". In summary, those with the financial means to buy more and/or better supplements will live longer. While it is difficult to argue that the advertising of supplements has created this sense of an inevitability regarding global and local health inequity, it is evident that supplement advertising reflects and re-enforces this sense of health inequity even while it purports to offer better health for the purchaser.

Conclusion: Supplements as a Foretaste of the Future?

> The more we become masters of our genetic endowments, the greater the burden we bear for the talents we have and the way we perform. Today when a basketball player misses a rebound, his coach can blame him for being out of position. Tomorrow the coach may blame him for being too short. Even now the use of performance-enhancing drugs in professional sports is subtly transforming the expectations players have for one another; on some teams players who take the field free from amphetamines or other stimulants are criticized for 'playing naked.' (Sandel 2004)

Sandel's hypothetical scenario suggests that in future we may be blamed for not taking the available substances or supplements that would otherwise rectify physical imperfections. This analysis suggests that while we have not reached the stage of blaming others for their physical or mental imperfections, we are already becoming conditioned to at least self-blame when we do not take steps to fully commit to being healthy. Moreover, we are gradually becoming accustomed to viewing a particular type of health—a health which augments capacities to above the norm—as desirable through the purchasing of supplement products. Using images and text which suggest supplement taking will augment physical and mental capacity, maintain and boost health, and ultimately differentiate ourselves as individuals from others in terms of health, supplement advertisers both reflect and encourage a version of health that is commercially oriented with little room for failure. If the advertising of supplements is suggestive of how we perceive health today and into the future, it is strongly suggestive of a society which is becoming conditioned to seeing health in competitive terms with the desire to over-achieve overriding collective and civil notions of health for all.

References

Agliata, D., & Tantleff-Dunn, S. (2004). The impact of media exposure on males' body image. *Journal of Social and Clinical Psychology, 23*(1), 7–22.

Alexander, S. M. (2003). Stylish hard bodies: Branded masculinity in Men's Health magazine. *Sociological Perspectives, 46*(4), 535–554.

Bailey, R. L., Gahche, J. J., Lentino, C. V., Dwyer, J. T., Engel, J. S., Thomas, P. R., et al. (2011). Dietary supplement use in the United States, 2003–2006. *The Journal of Nutrition, 141*(2), 261–266.

Banjo, O. C., Nadler, R., & Reiner, P. B. (2010). Physician attitudes towards pharmacological cognitive enhancement: Safety concerns are paramount. *PLoS One, 5*(12), e14322.

Bent, S. (2008). Herbal medicine in the United States: Review of efficacy, safety, and regulation. *Journal of General Internal Medicine, 23*(6), 854–859.

Blond, A. (2008). Impacts of exposure to images of ideal bodies on male body dissatisfaction: A review. *Body Image, 5*(3), 244–250.

Bolton, L. E., Cohen, J. B., & Bloom, P. N. (2006). Does marketing products as remedies create "get out of jail free cards"? *Journal of Consumer Research, 33*(1), 71–81.

Bolton, L. E., Reed II, A., Volpp, K. G., & Armstrong, K. (2008). How does drug and supplement marketing affect a healthy lifestyle? *Journal of Consumer Research, 34*(5), 713–726.

Bostrom, N., & Sandberg, A. (2009). Cognitive enhancement: Methods, ethics, regulatory challenges. *Science and Engineering Ethics, 15*(3), 311–341.

Botta, R. A. (2003). For your health? The relationship between magazine reading and adolescents' body image and eating disturbances. *Sex Roles, 48*(9–10), 389–399.

Bunton, R. (1997). Popular health, advanced liberalism and good housekeeping magazine. In R. Bunton & A. Petersen (Eds.), *Foucault, health and medicine*. London: Routledge.

Cakic, V. (2009). Smart drugs for cognitive enhancement: Ethical and pragmatic considerations in the era of cosmetic neurology. *Journal of Medical Ethics, 35*(10), 611–615.

Crawshaw, P. (2007). Governing the healthy male citizen: Men, masculinity and popular health in *Men's Health* magazine. *Social Science & Medicine, 65*(8), 1606–1618.

Cusumano, D. L., & Thompson, J. K. (1997). Body image and body shape ideals in magazines: Exposure, awareness, and internalization. *Sex Roles, 37*(9), 701–721.

Dascombe, B. J., Karunaratna, M., Cartoon, J., Fergie, B., & Goodman, C. (2010). Nutritional supplementation habits and perceptions of elite athletes within a state-based sporting institute. *Journal of Science and Medicine in Sport, 13*(2), 274–280.

DeLorme, D. E., Huh, J., Reid, L. N., & An, S. (2012). Dietary supplement advertising in the US. *International Journal of Advertising, 31*(3), 547–577.

Dickinson, A., Blatman, J., El-Dash, N., & Franco, J. C. (2014). Consumer usage and reasons for using dietary supplements: Report of a series of surveys. *Journal of the American College of Nutrition, 33*(2), 176–182.

Dworkin, S. L., & Wachs, F. L. (2009). *Body panic: Gender, health, and the selling of fitness*. New York: NYU Press.

Field, A. E., Austin, S. B., Camargo, C. A., Taylor, C. B., Striegel-Moore, R. H., Loud, K. J., et al. (2005). Exposure to the mass media, body shape concerns, and use of supplements to improve weight and shape among male and female adolescents. *Pediatrics, 116*(2), e214–e220.

Forlini, C., & Racine, E. (2009). Autonomy and coercion in academic "cognitive enhancement" using methylphenidate: Perspectives of key stakeholders. *Neuroethics, 2*(3), 163–177.

Gahche, J., Bailey, R., Burt, V., Hughes, J., Yetley, E., Dwyer, J., et al. (2011). Dietary supplement use among US adults has increased since NHANES III (1988–1994). *NCHS Data Brief, 61*, 1–8.

Garcia-Alvarez, A., Egan, B., de Klein, S., Dima, L., Maggi, F. M., Isoniemi, M., et al. (2014). Usage of plant food supplements across six european countries: Findings from the Plant LIBRA Consumer Survey. *PloS One, 9*(3), e92265.

Gough, B. (2006). Try to be healthy, but don't forgo your masculinity: Deconstructing men's health discourse in the media. *Social Science & Medicine, 63*(9), 2476–2488.

Greely, H., Sahakian, B., Harris, J., Kessler, R. C., Gazzaniga, M., Campbell, P., et al. (2008). Towards responsible use of cognitive-enhancing drugs by the healthy. *Nature, 456*(7223), 702–705.

Hargreaves, D. A., & Tiggemann, M. (2004). Idealized media images and adolescent body image: "Comparing" boys and girls. *Body Image, 1*(4), 351–361.

Hatoum, I. J., & Belle, D. (2004). Mags and abs: Media consumption and bodily concerns in men. *Sex Roles, 51*(7–8), 397–407.

Hemphill, D. (2009). Performance enhancement and drug control in sport: Ethical considerations. *Sport in Society, 12*(3), 313–326.

Henderson, S., & Petersen, A. R. (Eds.) (2002). *Consuming health: The commodification of health care.* London: Routledge.

Hotze, T. D., Shah, K., Anderson, E. E., & Wynia, M. K. (2011). "Doctor, would you prescribe a pill to help me…?" A national survey of physicians on using medicine for human enhancement. *American Journal of Bioethics, 11*(1), 3–13.

Kayser, B., Mauron, A., & Miah, A. (2007). Current anti-doping policy: A critical appraisal. *BMC medical ethics, 8*(1), 2.

Labre, M. P. (2005). The male body ideal: Perspectives of readers and non-readers of fitness magazines. *Journal of Men's Health and Gender, 2*(2), 223–229.

Larriviere, D., Williams, M. A., Rizzo, M., & Bonnie, R. J. (2009). Responding to requests from adult patients for neuroenhancements: Guidance of the Ethics, Law and Humanities Committee. *Neurology, 73*(17), 1406–1412.

Lucke, J., & Partridge, B. (2013). Towards a smart population: A public health framework for cognitive enhancement. *Neuroethics, 6*(2), 419–427.

Marik, P. E., & Flemmer, M. (2012). Do dietary supplements have beneficial health effects in industrialized nations what is the evidence? *Journal of Parenteral and Enteral Nutrition, 36*(2), 159–168.

Mason, M. J., & Scammon, D. L. (2000). Health claims and disclaimers: extended boundaries and research opportunities in consumer interpretation. *Journal of Public Policy & Marketing, 19*(1), 144–150.

Mason, M. J., & Scammon, D. L. (2011). Unintended consequences of health supplement information regulations: The importance of recognizing consumer motivations. *Journal of Consumer Affairs, 45*(2), 201–223.

McCabe, S. E., Knight, J. R., Teter, C. J., & Wechsler, H. (2005). Non-medical use of prescription stimulants among US college students: Prevalence and correlates from a national survey. *Addiction, 100*(1), 96–106.

Miah, A. (2007). Genetics, bioethics and sport. *Sports, Ethics and Philosophy*, *1*(2), 146–158.

Morgan, W. J. (2009). Athletic perfection, performance-enhancing drugs, and the treatment-enhancement distinction. *Journal of the Philosophy of Sport*, *36*(2), 162–181.

Morry, M. M., & Staska, S. L. (2001). Magazine exposure: Internalization, self-objectification, eating attitudes, and body satisfaction in male and female university students. *Canadian Journal of Behavioural Science*, *33*(4), 269–279.

Murphy, P., & Waddington, I. (1998). Sport for all: Some public health policy issues and problems. *Critical Public Health*, *8*(3), 193–205.

Nichter, M., & Thompson, J. J. (2006). For my wellness, not just my illness: North Americans' use of dietary supplements. *Culture, Medicine and Psychiatry*, *30*(2), 175–222.

Outram, S. M. (2013). Discourses of performance enhancement: Can we separate performance enhancement from performance enhancing drug use? *Performance Enhancement & Health*, *2*(3), 94–100.

Parens, E. (1998). Is better always good?: The enhancement project. *Hastings Center Report*, *28*(1), s1–s17.

Parens, E. (2005). Authenticity and ambivalence: Toward understanding the enhancement debate. *Hastings Center Report*, *35*(3), 34–41.

Persson, I., & Savulescu, J. (2008). The perils of cognitive enhancement and the urgent imperative to enhance the moral character of humanity. *Journal of Applied Philosophy*, *25*(3), 162–177.

Petróczi, A., & Aidman, E. (2008). Psychological drivers in doping: the lifecycle model of performance enhancement. *Substance Abuse Treatment, Prevention, and Policy*, *3*(1). doi:10.1186/1747-597X-3-.

Pomeranz, J. L., Barbosa, G., Killian, C., & Austin, S. B. (2014). The dangerous mix of adolescents and dietary supplements for weight loss and muscle building: Legal strategies for state action. *Journal of Public Health Management and Practice*, 1–8.

Quinones, R. L., Winsor, R. D., Patino, A., & Hoffmann, P. (2013). The regulation of dietary supplements within the united states: Flawed attempts at mending a defective consumer safety mechanism. *Journal of Consumer Affairs*, *47*(2), 328–357.

Reinert, A., Rohrmann, S., Becker, N., & Linseisen, P. D. J. (2007). Lifestyle and diet in people using dietary supplements. *European Journal of Nutrition*, *46*(3), 165–173.

Ritchie, M. (2007). Use of herbal supplements and nutritional supplements in the UK: What do we know about their pattern of usage? *Proceedings of the Nutrition Society, 66*(4), 479–482.

Rotfeld, H. J. (2009). Health information consumers can't or don't want to use. *Journal of Consumer Affairs, 43*(2), 373–377.

Rose, N. (2001). The politics of life itself. *Theory, Culture & Society, 18*(6), 1–30.

Sandel, M. (2004). The case against perfection. *The Atlantic Monthly, 293*(3), 50–62.

Schermer, M. (2008). On the argument that enhancement is "cheating". *Journal of Medical Ethics, 34*(2), 85–88.

Simon, R. L. (1984). Good competition and drug-enhanced performance. *Journal of the Philosophy of Sport, 11*(1), 6–13.

Smith, A. C., & Stewart, B. (2008). Drug policy in sport: Hidden assumptions and inherent contradictions. *Drug and Alcohol Review, 27*(2), 123–129.

Stibbe, A. (2004). Health and the social construction of masculinity in Men's Health magazine. *Men and Masculinities, 7*(1), 31–51.

Thompson, J. J., & Nichter, M. (2007). The compliance paradox: What we need to know about "real-world" dietary supplement use in the United States. *Alternative Therapies in Health and Medicine, 13*(2), 48–55.

Tiggemann, M., & McGill, B. (2004). The role of social comparison in the effect of magazine advertisements on women's mood and body dissatisfaction. *Journal of Social and Clinical Psychology, 23*(1), 23–44.

WADA. (2015). *Anti-Doping Code 2015* (p. 30). Accessed January 5, 2015, from https://wada-main-prod.s3.amazonaws.com/resources/files/wada-2015-world-anti-doping-code.pdf

Waddington, I., Malcolm, D., & Green, K. (1997). Sport, health and physical education: A reconsideration. *European Physical Education Review, 3*(2), 165–182.

Wolpe, P. R. (2002). Treatment, enhancement, and the ethics of neurotherapeutics. *Brain and Cognition, 50*(3), 387–395.

7

Smoking and Appearance

Sarah Grogan

Context

Currently around 9.4 million adults in the UK are regular cigarette smokers, and smoking kills more than 100,000 people in the UK each year (Cancer Research UK 2015). Smoking is thought to be directly responsible for around 90 % of lung cancer deaths in the USA, as well as being a major cause of coronary heart disease and stroke (American Lung Association 2015; NHS 2015a). Lung cancer rates are increasing in women in the UK, and lung cancer now kills more women each year than breast cancer (NHS 2015b).

In spite of health promotion campaigns designed to reduce smoking, 22 % men and 19 % women in the UK (Cancer Research UK 2015), and 21 % men and 16 % women in the USA (Centers for Disease Control and Prevention 2013) are regular smokers. The prevalence of tobacco use is highest in young adults in both the USA and the UK. In the UK the

---

S. Grogan (✉)
Department of Psychology, Manchester Metropolitan University,
53, Bonsall Street, Manchester, M156GX, UK

© The Editor(s) (if applicable) and The Author(s) 2016
M. Hall et al. (eds.), *Chemically Modified Bodies*,
DOI 10.1057/978-1-137-53535-1_7

highest incidence for women is amongst 25–34-year-olds, where 27.8 % of men and 19.8 % of women are regular smokers (Cancer Research UK 2015). In the UK, two-thirds of smokers start to smoke before the age of 18 (Action on Smoking and Health 2015), and in 2012, 23 % of adolescents in England had tried cigarettes, and 4 % were smoking at least one cigarette a week (Health and Social Care Information Centre 2013). In the USA, 6.7 % of middle school and 23.3 % of high school students smoke (Centers for Disease Control and Prevention 2014).

The nicotine in cigarettes is usually identified as the key factor in addiction to cigarette smoking. However, psychological factors are also important in initiation and maintenance of smoking. In focus groups carried out in the UK, young men and women reported that they felt under considerable social pressure to initiate and maintain smoking, and felt they needed to provide excuses such as having asthma or needing to be fit for playing sport to be able to refuse cigarettes and still be accepted by their peer groups (Fry et al. 2009; Gough et al. 2009). Smoking seems to be subject to social context, and psychological factors are implicated in both uptake and maintenance of smoking.

Body Weight and Smoking

Women smokers tend to have a lower body mass index (BMI) and smaller waist circumference than those who have never smoked (Kaufman et al. 2012). Nicotine tends to suppress appetite, and smoking reduces palatability of food through reductions in taste and smell (Mineur et al. 2011). Smoking can also be a distraction from eating. Most people gain weight on quitting smoking when appetite and metabolic rate revert to pre-smoking levels, food becomes more palatable, and smoking is no longer a viable distraction from eating (Williamson et al. 1991), although levels of sedentary activity may also play a role in weight gain in smokers who quit (Kaufman et al. 2012).

Weight concern may be crucial in the decision to smoke or to quit, and qualitative work has shown that women smokers report initiating smoking to reduce appetite and to assist in dieting (Grogan et al. 2009). There is also good evidence from quantitative studies that young women may use smoking as a way to reduce appetite, to help with weight loss diets and to maintain current weight (e.g. Potter et al. 2004). Women who smoke tend to endorse thinner ideal body sizes than women who do not smoke (Pomerleau and Saules (2007) and are more likely than non-smokers to use unsafe weight loss practices such as diet pills and fasting to lose weight (Stice and Shaw 2003). Smoking is adopted by people who are weight concerned to reduce appetite and aid in weight loss, and concern about gaining weight may be a significant disincentive for quitting smoking.

Body Image and Smoking

Cross-Sectional Studies

Body dissatisfaction has been reliably linked to smoking and cross-sectional studies, which measure body satisfaction in smokers and non-smokers, tend to find female smokers are less satisfied with their bodies than non-smokers (Grogan et al. 2010a; Grogan 2012). Most research linking body satisfaction with smoking has focused on women smokers, and there are very few studies of men's body satisfaction related to smoking. However, there is some evidence that male smokers may be less body satisfied than non-smokers (Grogan et al. 2010a), suggesting similar links between smoking and body satisfaction to those found in women. Women smokers also tend to endorse a thinner ideal body than non-smokers. Pomerleau and Saules (2007) compared 420 women who were current smokers with 167 never-smokers and found that smokers endorsed a thinner ideal body shape and scored significantly lower on a single-item measure of body satisfaction ("I am satisfied with the shape of my body"). In one interesting study, women smokers were found to be more likely to report being ashamed of their bodies and to monitor them for faults than women who had never smoked (Fissel and Lafreniere 2006). Although the cross-sectional nature of this study does not enable us to determine whether self-objectification causes smoking, it does suggest important links between women's self-objectification and smoking.

Longitudinal Work

One of the ways to interrogate directional pathways between body dissatisfaction and smoking is to measure these variables over time. King et al. (2005) carried out a prospective US study where body image was measured before quitting smoking. They showed that both body dissatisfaction and perception of body size were important predictors of smoking outcomes at the end of a 12-week randomized smoking cessation trial. Women smokers who had a greater discrepancy between actual and ideal size, and those who over-estimated their body size had most difficulty quitting smoking. The authors conclude that women who feel overweight may use smoking to try to control their eating. They also suggest that women who experience psychological distress related to their perception of being overweight may use smoking to help them to cope with this distress, and that body dissatisfaction precedes smoking. The authors also investigated whether quitting smoking would impact body image and found that body dissatisfaction increased in women who quit smoking on their programme. Once increases in weight gain were controlled for, there were no significant changes in body dissatisfaction in those who had quit smoking, showing that changes in body satisfaction following smoking cessation are likely to be the result of weight gain on quitting smoking.

Experimental Studies

Another useful way to determine temporal relationships between body image and smoking is to manipulate body image and investigate impact on smoking-related attitudes and behaviours. Experimental studies have tended to find that interventions designed to increase weight concerns promote increases in smoking, supporting the idea that appearance concerns precede smoking. Lopez et al. (2008) exposed women smokers aged 18–24 years to thin body image cues and smoking cues and investigated women's urge for cigarettes. They found that increasing women's weight concern experimentally through presentation of thin model images increased their urge to smoke. Interestingly, women higher in initial weight dissatisfaction were most affected by the thin model images in the absence of smoking cues. They conclude that the main effect of the thin-model manipulation, added to the moderating effect of trait weight satisfaction, is evidence for a causal role of weight concern on smoking motivation. The effect was not moderated by women's body mass index, suggesting that it was women's subjective weight rather than their actual weight that influenced their urge to smoke in response to the thin models. The authors suggest that perception of overweight seems to be a greater motivator for smoking than actual size.

Lopez et al.'s (2008) study was very well controlled and one of the few studies to date to actually manipulate weight concern in women smokers and observe the direct impact on their smoking behaviour. It showed that weight dissatisfaction can lead to smoking, at least in the highly controlled conditions utilized in this study, and that weight dissatisfaction may precede smoking rather than vice versa. It does not address the question of whether some other factor, such as negative affect or self-esteem, explains the relationship between seeing the model images and smoking or whether there is a direct relationship such that women see the images and smoke in the expectation that smoking will control their weight. Qualitative work shows that women report using smoking self-consciously to control their weight and that both men and women see smoking as a viable weight-control strategy for women (Grogan et al. 2009). This means that the direct path, where smoking is taken up specifically to reduce weight seems feasible, although further quantitative work is needed in this area to study potential mediating pathways and impacts of other variables. However, it is clear from this study that reducing weight concerns in women may be a useful way to reduce smoking, and the authors suggest that weight concerns should be the direct targets of interventions to help women to quit smoking.

Relatively few studies have investigated systematically what happens to smoking when weight concerns are *reduced* in samples of smokers (Flett et al. 2012). However, in one study that has tackled this issue, Perkins et al. (2001) found some evidence that interventions designed to reduce weight concerns may help women quit smoking. As part of a smoking cessation programme with women smokers in the USA who were concerned about weight gain, women were educated about the amount of weight most women might expect to gain when quitting smoking and the fact that it is healthier to gain a bit of weight than to continue to smoke. They were also taught to challenge negative thoughts about their bodies, dieting was discouraged, and women were taught about healthy eating. This intervention produced significantly higher smoking abstinence rates than a condition where women discussed non-weight-related aspects of smoking such as impact on their families, and a programme where women were taught about diet and exercise as ways to control weight. The authors conclude that interventions designed to reduce weight concerns can improve smoking cessation outcome in weight-concerned women for up to one year post intervention. In another similar study, Copeland et al. (2006) focused on whether advice on reducing weight concerns should be individually tailored or could be generic. In their study, weight-concerned US women smokers allocated to an individually tailored programme had significantly better smoking abstinence rates at three months and six months post treatment than those in a general feedback condition. This suggests that addressing specific weight concerns with individual women, rather than giving generic guidance on reducing weight concerns, can be important in preventing relapse into smoking.

We still need to know much more about appearance concerns and smoking in men, and about what happens when appearance concerns are reduced in men as all intervention work to date focuses on women. There has been an assumption in previous work that men are not concerned about weight gain on quitting smoking. Although previous work suggests that men may be less concerned than women about weight gain on quitting smoking (Grogan et al. 2009), this may be a concern for some men and should not be overlooked. Reducing such concerns may be an effective way to enable some men to reduce smoking.

Facial Ageing and Smoking

In addition to issues around body image, women (and men) may be concerned that smoking will age their skin, especially on the face. Smokers tend to develop more wrinkles earlier in life as nicotine ingestion narrows blood vessels, impairing blood flow to the skin. This reduces uptake of oxygen and vitamin A, and chemicals in tobacco smoke may also damage collagen and elastin fibres, so that skin wrinkles prematurely (Helfrich et al. 2007; Vierkötter and Krutmann 2012). Since the Western ideal is smooth skin with minimal wrinkles, particularly for women, this may deter people from smoking. Focus groups with 87 UK men and women between 17 and 24 years old asking about the impacts of smoking on how people looked (Grogan et al. 2009), found that women non-smokers were very concerned about skin ageing. In this study, male and female smokers were very concerned about having clear skin without visible wrinkles and said that they would definitely quit if their skin started to show the effects of smoking. None of these young smokers had experienced any obvious impacts on their skin of smoking and most did not believe that skin-ageing was a realistic and self-relevant risk for them personally. This meant that they did not intend to quit at the time when they were interviewed.

One way to highlight self-relevance of negative impacts of smoking on appearance is to show realistic images of the likely effect that smoking will have on an individual's face. This has recently become possible through the development of sophisticated computer techniques such as age-progression software. Developments in software have now made it possible to show the differential effects of not smoking versus smoking achieved through using wrinkling/ageing algorithms based on photographs of groups of smokers and on published data relating to specific effects on the skin produced by smoking. Using these age-progression techniques, a digital photograph is altered to show how his or her own face would be likely to age with and without smoking.

Studies of the effectiveness of these kinds of programmes are producing promising results. In one such study, young women smokers aged 18–34 years exposed to an age-appearance morphing intervention were very concerned about the impact of ageing on their faces in general, and in particular the additional impact of smoking on their skin (Grogan et al. 2010b). In this study, women reported that seeing their own face aged on the computer screen had convinced them that they were at risk of skin wrinkling if they continued to smoke, and that they were highly motivated to quit smoking as a result of the intervention. Many reported that they would take active steps to quit having seen how they would look if they continued to smoke.

Randomized controlled trials have also shown that exposure to age-progression facial morphing can impact on smoking-related attitudes and behaviour. One study investigated whether exposure to the facial age-progression technique impacted on quit smoking cognitions, nicotine dependence, and self-reported and objectively assessed smoking in 70 young women smokers (Grogan et al. 2011). Women completed questionnaires assessing quit smoking attitudes, subjective norms, perceived behavioural control and intention immediately before, immediately after, and four weeks after receiving the intervention or usual care. At the first and last time points they also completed measures of nicotine dependence, self-reported and objectively assessed smoking (breath carbon monoxide levels). Women in the appearance-related intervention condition had significantly more positive quit smoking attitudes, norms, perceived behavioural control, and intentions immediately after exposure compared to controls. Only the effects on quit smoking attitudes remained significant at four weeks post-intervention. Nicotine dependence and self-reported smoking (cigarettes per week), but not objective smoking, were significantly lower in the intervention compared to control group at four weeks. The results of these two studies suggest that age-appearance facial morphing may be useful in smoking cessation programmes with young women smokers.

Work conducted thus far suggests that age-appearance morphing techniques may be effective in helping women to take active steps to quit smoking. Further work is ongoing to look at the effectiveness of these kinds of techniques with male smokers. Work with young men shows generally positive impacts on motivation to quit smoking, although some men have been found to be unconcerned about skin ageing (Flett et al. 2015) supporting facial morphing research where young men have been shown impacts of UV protection on their skin (Williams et al. 2013a). It is important to understand more about the likely impacts of these kinds of techniques with male smokers. It is also important to understand how to maintain the effectiveness of these interventions and work is ongoing to investigate what kinds of materials and messages might be helpful in doing this. It is also crucial to understand whether these kinds of techniques are particularly effective for particular groups of women or men, for instance those who are more heavily invested in their appearance. Also, women smokers have reported stress and physiological arousal at seeing the damage that smoking is likely to be doing to their skin, possibly the result of cognitive dissonance between smoking behaviour and potential negative outcomes (Grogan et al. 2010b). It will be interesting to see whether this self-reported arousal can be picked up using physiological measures, and whether arousal levels predict attitudinal and behaviour change following the intervention. All this work is ongoing and all important in developing our understanding of the benefits of facial morphing techniques in changing smoking-related attitudes and behaviours.

Implications for Healthcare Practice

Smoking Cessation

Data presented earlier showing that both men and women smokers have increased body dissatisfaction, and that women smokers have increased body shame and weight concern, suggests that health practitioners who want to reduce smoking need to pay serious consideration to finding ways of reducing appearance-related concerns as a way to reduce smoking. There is certainly potential for reducing smoking in women who already smoke through reducing weight concerns. Raising specific appearance concerns by showing people how their face will look when they are older if they continue to smoke may also be an effective way to reduce smoking. However, raising appearance concerns may also promote lowered self-esteem. O'Dea (2012) has shown that lowered self-esteem is closely associated with negative body image and may result in the elevation of other negative health behaviours such as extreme dieting and use of performance-enhancing drugs which are both associated with low self-esteem. So although smoking may be reduced, other negative health behaviours may be increased unless careful debriefing is carried out to ensure that participants do not become generally more concerned about their appearance after the intervention. Work using body-acceptance strategies such as suggested by Tylka (2011) may be helpful in reducing any potential negative impacts, and are also likely to boost body image and reduce weight concerns. Any such interventions need to be administered with care by people who are aware of the possible negative impacts, to promote self-efficacy related to quitting smoking. This will ensure that smokers are clear that they will avoid the negative impact of smoking on their skin if they quit, promoting accountability and placing responsibility with them to make the choice as to how they wish to look in the future.

Smoking Initiation

According to Action on Smoking and Health, adolescent smoking in the UK is a significant health problem, with two-thirds of smokers starting to smoke before the age of 18 (Action on Smoking and Health 2015) although it is illegal to sell cigarettes to anyone under 18 in the UK. Appearance is a key concern for adolescents in the UK, and girls are also generally more concerned about their appearance (Grogan 2008; Grogan et al. 2014), so focussing on the negative impacts of smoking on appearance may be a useful way to enable girls in particular to resist smoking their first cigarette.

There is very little work in this area, although Hysert et al. (2003) found that when adolescents were shown impacts of smoking on other people's faces, they showed significantly more negative attitudes to smoking on the questions, "Do you think that people risk harming themselves if they smoke one or less than one cigarette per day?" and "Does concern about your appearance affect the choices you make from day to day?" This demonstrates that showing non-smokers the differential impacts of smoking on facial ageing can impact on their attitudes towards smoking. Work in the UK has also shown that facial ageing interventions can be effective in changing male and female adolescents' views of health behaviours such as suntanning (Williams et al. 2013b) and that both male and female adolescents are concerned about skin damage caused by health-related behaviours (Williams et al. 2013c), suggesting that age-progression morphing techniques might also be effective in smoking prevention work.

There is still a lot of work to be done in determining how to produce effective, gender- and age-specific interventions that use appearance concerns to prevent smoking initiation in non-smokers, although UK work where adolescents have been shown other people's faces morphed, and UK work on tanning where adolescents have had their own faces morphed, suggests that this might be possible using age-progression software. If these strategies are to be incorporated into children's education they need to be discussed with children and parents from these target groups, and delivered by practitioners who are seen as credible to the children involved, so that they seem meaningful to young people in this age range. Interventions also need to be conducted in ways that avoid raising additional appearance concerns, using strategic debriefing to ensure that children understand that if they do not start smoking they do not need to worry about the ageing effects of smoking on their skin. Work on facial morphing and tanning with adolescents can perhaps be used to enable researchers to ensure that interventions will be meaningful to adolescent girls and boys who may not yet have smoked their first cigarette.

Summary

Tobacco use remains high in young men and women in the UK and elsewhere, and work reviewed here suggests that smoking is associated with poor body image. This makes it similar to other health-risking behaviours such as sun exposure without sunblock which have also been linked with low appearance evaluation (Blashill et al. 2015). Smoking is linked (especially for women smokers) with weight concern, and research data suggests that interventions focusing on reducing concerns about weight gain may be effective in enabling women smokers to quit. Concerns about facial appearance are relevant to the decision whether to quit smoking in both men and women, and smoking-related interventions focusing specifically on facial appearance may be useful for both genders to avoid smoking initiation and to enable smokers to quit smoking.

Although evidence suggests some important links between appearance concerns and smoking, there is still a lot of work to be done to clarify the nature of these associations. We need to know much more about the impacts of reducing weight concerns in male smokers, and links between facial ageing concerns and smoking in older men and women. Also, now that e-cigarette use is increasing in the UK (Dockrell et al. 2013; Brown et al. 2014) we need to understand more about the links between body weight, weight concern, and use of e-cigarettes. Evidence that concern about weight gain may be an important disincentive for quitting smoking may be useful information for those trying to encourage people to switch, particularly if smoking e-cigarettes enables smokers to control their weight. In particular, we need to be sure that all interventions are delivered by trained and empathic practitioners to ensure that they promote quitting, or avoidance of smoking initiation, without increasing appearance dissatisfaction in people who may already have concerns in this area.

References

Action on Smoking and Health. (2014). *Fact sheet: Young people and smoking.* Accessed March 24, 2015, from www.ash.org.uk/files/documents/ASH_108.pdf

Action on Smoking and Health. (2015). *Smoking statistics.* Accessed March 5, 2015, from http://www.ash.org.uk/information/facts-and-stats/fact-sheets

American Lung Association. (2015). *Smoking.* Accessed March 5, 2015, from http://www.lung.org/stop-smoking/about-smoking/health-effects/smoking.html

Blashill, A., Williams, A., Grogan, S., & Clark-Carter, D. (2015). Negative appearance evaluation is associated with skin cancer risk behaviors among American men and women. *Health Psychology, 34*(1), 93–96.

Brown, J., West, R., Beard, E., Michie, S., Shahab, L., & McNeill, A. (2014). Prevalence and characteristics of e-cigarette users in Great Britain: Findings from a general population survey of smokers. *Addictive Behaviour, 39,* 1120–1125.

Cancer Research UK (2015). *Tobacco statistics.* Accessed March 5, 2015, from http://www.cancerresearchuk.org/cancer-info/cancerstats/causes/tobacco-statistics/

Cash, T. (2000) *Users manuals for the multidimensional body-self relations questionnaire*. Available from the author on http://www.body-images.com

Centers for Disease Control and Prevention. (2013). *Smoking*. Accessed March 4, 2015, from http://www.cdc.gov/nchs/fastats/smoking.htm

Centers for Disease Control and Prevention. (2014). *Youth and tobacco use*. Accessed March 1, 2015, from http://www.cdc.gov/tobacco/data_statistics/fact_sheets/youth_data/tobacco_use/index.htm

Copeland, A. L., Martin, P. D., Geiselman, P. J., Rash, C. J., & Kendzor, D. E. (2006). Smoking cessation for weight-concerned women: Group vs. individually tailored, dietary, and weight-control follow-up sessions. *Addictive Behaviors, 31*, 115–127.

Croghan, I. T., Bronars, C., Patten, C. A., Schroeder, D. R., Nirelli, L. M., Thomas, J. L., Clark, M. M., Vickers, K. S., Foraker, R., Lane, K., Houlihan, D., Offord, K. P., & Hurt, R. D. (2006). Is smoking related to body image satisfaction, stress, and self-esteem in young adults? *American Journal of Health Behavior, 30*, 322–333.

Dockrell, M., Morison, R., Bauld, L., & McNeill, A. (2013). E-cigarettes: Prevalence and attitudes in Great Britain. *Nicotine Tobacco Research, 15*, 1737–1744.

Fissel, D. L., & Lafreniere, K. D. (2006). Weight control motives for cigarette smoking: Further consequences of the sexual objectification of women? *Feminism and Psychology, 16*, 327–344.

Flett, K., Clark-Carter, D., Grogan, S., & Davey, R. (2012). How effective are physical appearance interventions in changing smoking perceptions, attitudes and behaviours? A systematic review. *Tobacco Control*. doi:10.1136/tobaccocontrol-2011-050236.

Flett, K., Grogan, S., Clark-Carter, D., Gough, B., & Conner, M. (2015). Male smokers' experiences of an appearance-focused facial-ageing intervention. *Journal of Health Psychology*. doi:10.1177/1359105315603477.

Fredrickson, B. L., & Roberts, T. A. (1997). Objectification theory: Toward understanding women's lived experiences and mental health risks. *Psychology of Women Quarterly, 21*, 173–206.

Fry, G., Grogan, S., Gough, B., & Conner, M. (2009). Smoking in the lived world: How young people make sense of the social role cigarettes play in their lives. *British Journal of Social Psychology, 47*, 763–780.

Gough, B., Fry, G., Grogan, S., & Conner, M. (2009). Why do young adult smokers continue to smoke despite the health risks? A focus group study. *Psychology and Health, 24*, 203–220.

Grogan, S. (2008). *Body image: Understanding body dissatisfaction in men, women and children* (2nd ed.). New York: Routledge.

Grogan, S. (2012). Smoking and body image. In T. Cash (Ed.), *Encyclopedia of body image and human appearance* (pp. 745–750). London: Elsevier.

Grogan, S., Fry, G., Gough, B., & Conner, M. (2009). Smoking to stay thin or giving up to save face. Young men and women talk about appearance concerns and smoking. *British Journal of Health Psychology, 14*, 175–186.

Grogan, S., Hartley, L., Fry, G., Conner, M., & Gough, B. (2010a). Appearance concerns and smoking in young men and women: going beyond weight control. *Drugs: Education, Prevention and Policy, 17*, 261–269.

Grogan, S., Flett, K., Clark-Carter, D., Gough, B., Davey, R., Richardson, D., & Rajaratnam, G. (2010b). 'Women smokers' experiences of an age-appearance anti-smoking intervention: A qualitative study. *British Journal of Health Psychology, 16*, 675–689.

Grogan, S., Flett, K., Clark-Carter, D., Conner, M., Davey, R., Richardson, D., & Rajaratnam, G. (2011). A randomized controlled trial of an appearance-related smoking intervention. *Health Psychology, 6*, 805–809.

Grogan, S., Williams, A., Kilgariff, S., Bunce, J., Heyland, S. J., Padilla, T., et al. (2014). Dance and body image: Young people's experiences of a dance movement psychotherapy session. *Qualitative Research in Sport, Exercise and Health, 6*, 261–277.

Health and Social Care Information Centre. (2013). *Statistics on smoking, England—2013*. Accessed March 5, 2015, from http://www.hscic.gov.uk/catalogue/PUB11454

Helfrich, Y. R., Yu, L., Ofori, A., Hamilton, T. A., Lambert, J., King, A., Voorhees, J. J., & Kang, S. (2007). Effect of smoking on aging of photoprotected skin: Evidence gathered using a new photonumeric scale. *Archives of Dermatology, 143*, 397–402.

Hysert, P. E., Mirand, A. L., Giovino, G. A., Cummings, K. M., & Kuo, C. L. (2003). "At face value": Age progression software provides personalized demonstration of the effects of smoking on appearance (Letter). *Tobacco Control, 12*, 238.

Kaufman, A., Augustson, E. M., & Patrick, H. (2012). Unraveling the relationship between smoking and weight: The role of sedentary behavior. *Journal of Obesity, 2012*, 735465.

King, T. K., Matacin, M., White, K. S., & Marcus, B. H. (2005). A prospective examination of body image and smoking in women. *Body Image: An International Journal of Research, 2*, 19–28.

Lopez, E. N., Drobes, D. J., Thompson, J. K., & Brandon, T. H. (2008). Effects of a body image challenge on smoking motivation among college females. *Health Psychology, 27*, 243–251.

Mineur, Y. S., Abizaid, A., Rao, Y., Salas, R., DiLeone, R. J., D. Gündisch, et al. (2011) Nicotine decreases food intake through activation of POMC neurons. *Science, 332*, 1330–1332.

National Health Service. (2015a). *What are the health risks of smoking?* Accessed March 1, 2015, from http://www.nhs.uk/chq/Pages/2344.aspx?CategoryID=53andSubCategoryID=536

National Health Service. (2015b). *Lung cancer in women.* Accessed March 5, 2015, from http://www.nhs.uk/Livewell/Lungcancer/Pages/Womenandlungcancer.aspx

O'Dea, J. (2012). Body image and self-esteem. In T. Cash (Ed.), *Encyclopedia of body image and human appearance* (pp. 141–148). London: Elsevier.

Perkins, K. A., Marcus, M. D., Levine, M. D., D'Amico, D., Miller, A., Broge, M., et al. (2001). Cognitive behavioral therapy to reduce weight concerns improves smoking cessation outcome in weight-concerned women. *Journal of Consulting and Clinical Psychology, 69*, 604–613.

Pomerleau, C. S., & Saules, K. (2007). Body image, body satisfaction, and eating patterns in normal-weight and overweight/obese women current smokers and never-smokers. *Addictive Behaviours, 32*, 2329–2334.

Potter, B., Pederson, L. L., Chan, S. S. H., Aubut, J. L., & Koval, J. J. (2004). Does a relationship exist between body weight, concerns about weight, and smoking among adolescents? An integration of the literature with an emphasis on gender. *Nicotine and Tobacco Research, 6*, 397–425.

Stice, E., & Shaw, H. (2003). Prospective relations of body image, eating and affective disturbances to smoking onset in adolescent girls: How Virginia slims. *Journal of Consulting and Clinical Psychology, 71*, 129–135.

Tylka, T. L. (2011). Positive psychology perspectives on body image. In T. Cash & L. Smolak (Eds.), *Body image: A handbook of science, practice, and prevention* (pp. 56–64). New York: Guilford.

Vierkötter, A., & Krutmann, J. (2012). Environmental influences on skin aging and ethnic-specific manifestations. *Dermato-Endocrinology, 4*(3), 227–231. doi:10.4161/derm.19858.

Williams, A. L., Grogan, S., Buckley, E., & Clark-Carter, D. (2013a). Men's experiences of an appearance-focussed facial-ageing sun protection intervention: A qualitative study. *Body Image: An International Journal of Research, 10*, 263–266.

Williams, A. L., Grogan, S., Buckley, E., & Clark-Carter, D. (2013b). British adolescents' experiences of an appearance-focussed facial-ageing sun protection intervention: A qualitative study. *Education and Health, 31*, 97–101.

Williams, A., Grogan, S., Clark-Carter, D., & Buckley, E. (2013c). British adolescents' sun protection and UV exposure awareness. *British Journal of School Nursing, 8*, 436–441.

Williamson, D. F., Madans, J., Anda, R. F., Kleinman, J. C., Giovino, G. A., & Byers, T. (1991). Smoking cessation and severity of weight gain in a national cohort. *New England Journal of Medicine, 324*, 739–745.

8

Bodybuilders' Accounts of Synthol Use: The Construction of Lay Expertise

Matthew Hall, Sarah Grogan, and Brendan Gough

Introduction

Synthol is an injectable site-enhancement oil comprising 85 % oil (often sesame), 7.5 % lidocaine (a local anaesthetic) and 7.5 % alcohol (steriliser). Site-enhancement oils were developed at the start of the twentieth century, originally for use in cosmetic procedures such as breast augmentation and wrinkle reduction (Di Benedetto et al. 2002). More recently, synthol has been used by elite and lay bodybuilders to produce the cosmetic appearance of trained muscle (Childs 2007; Ghandourah et al. 2012).

M. Hall (✉)
Associate Academic, University of Derby, Department of Psychology, Kedleston Road, Derby DE22 1GB, UK

S. Grogan
Department of Psychology, Manchester Metropolitan University, Bonsall Street 53, M15 6GX, Manchester, UK

B. Gough
School of Social, Psychological and Communication Sciences, Leeds Beckett University, Calverly Building [Rm 919], City Campus, LS1 9HE, Leeds, UK

© The Editor(s) (if applicable) and The Author(s) 2016
M. Hall et al. (eds.), *Chemically Modified Bodies*,
DOI 10.1057/978-1-137-53535-1_8

Synthol is injected directly into muscle, where it causes swelling and enlargement, and is often used by bodybuilders to inflate one target muscle that is seen as out of proportion to the rest of the trained body (sometimes known as 'fluffing'; Childs 2007). It may also be used in large quantities by both experienced and the relatively inexperienced in order to develop all key muscles, leading to the appearance of a muscular body developed through weight training. However, perceived differences between these cosmetically enhanced body parts and those produced through weight training alone have been deemed "comically obvious" within the bodybuilding community, with "unnatural-appearing lumps" in muscles (Brainium 2013) framed as "freakish" and "bizarre" by bodybuilders who choose not to use synthol (Childs 2007).

Although medical evidence for negative effects of synthol is not well documented, there are many case reports citing complications in patients following injections of paraffin, sesame, and walnut oil, linking to stroke and pulmonary embolism, localized skin problems such as nerve damage and oil filled cysts, and muscle damage (Banke et al. 2012; Darsow et al. 2000). In one of the rare case studies of a bodybuilder using synthol, use was linked to complications such as muscle pain and muscular fibrosis (excessive formation of fibrous bands of scar tissue between muscle fibers; Ghandourah et al. 2012). So although synthol may give bodybuilders a way to rectify perceived shortcomings in particular muscles or muscle groups, it has been suggested that use destroys the injected muscle and may produce severe long-term health consequences (Brainium 2013; Ghandourah et al. 2012).

Synthol is widely available, and seems to be becoming more popular in the 2000s (Brainium 2013; Childs 2007). It may be attractive to some bodybuilders who may believe that it does not cause some of the more severe side effects linked with anabolic steroid use (Ghandourah et al. 2012); although others may see synthol use as risky and pointless as it does not lead to realistic-appearing muscle development (e.g. Brainium 2013). Reasons for continued use are poorly understood, and to our knowledge there are no published studies which examine how users talk to each other about their practices. Nearly two decades ago, Epstein (1995) pointed out in his study of AIDS activism that where there is an absence of specialist knowledge this gap is often filled with lay expertise.

Whilst some specialist knowledge on synthol exists (e.g. Darsow et al. 2000; Di Benedetto et al. 2002; Ghandourah et al. 2012), this information tends to be presented in academic publications not widely accessible to those outside academia (e.g. *International Journal of Sports Medicine*). In the context of this knowledge vacuum, we focus on how lay expertise is worked up by Internet forum contributors in order to be able to provide each other with support and advice.[1] Since posts are constructed by unknown others a key question emerges: how are forum contributors taken seriously? (Richardson 2003, p. 172). Epstein (1995) argues that this rests on five key elements: credibility, legitimation and trust, which allow for the provision of support and influence. It is these aspects that form the framework of our analysis.

Method

Data Collection

Synthol is widely available on the Internet as 'Pump and Pose' intramuscular injection oil. It has become "one of the most controversial in modern BB'ing" (Arnold 2014, p. 1) and arguably elsewhere too (e.g. *Amazon* reviews). Given the apparent controversy surrounding synthol we were not surprised to find very few people openly talking about its use. The few who have spoken about it in mainstream outlets such as *Amazon* customer feedback and *YouTube* responses tend to be met with responses such as:

> 5 stars if you are too lazy to work for what you don't deserve and need to inject jet fuel into your "muscles". If you are a tiny wuss that needs to look big without giving any effort to work out then this is surely for you. Shame on all of you who use this stuff, it is extremely unhealthy so you get what you deserve. (Amazon.com 2014: http://www.amazon.com/Synthol-posing-oil-100mil-bottles/dp/B00B0F3FAG/ref=pd_rhf_cr_p_img_1)

---

[1] Lay expertise may also be referred to as "broscience" (see http://broscience.co.uk/category/news/).

Indeed, the vast majority of *Google* hits portray users as having "comically obvious" and "unnatural-appearing" muscles (Brainium 2013; Childs 2007). Many of these were in response to apparent synthol misuse (e.g. Moustafa Ismail, who currently holds the Guinness Book of Records for 31″ arms). Those who did talk about their synthol use tended to be elite bodybuilders (e.g. USA championship winner Rich Piana). Given their use can be framed as a professional requirement, we focussed instead on a unique forum thread where lay bodybuilders discussed their usage. Seventeen self-identified bodybuilders contributed to the AlinBoard: Anabolic Steroid Discussion Forum thread "Did My First Shots of Synthol Today!!!!" the main thrust of which was from July to September 2006 (as of 20 August 2014).

Founded in 2003 *AllinShop* claims to be the largest Internet overseas pharmacy and a "professional IFBB[2] supplier". In particular, *AllinShop* supplies elite and non-elite bodybuilders ergogenic[3] drugs such as steroids (Anavar, Dianabol, Sustanon 250), β-agonists (e.g. clenbuterol), hormones (e.g. human growth hormone, thyroxine) and other adrenal hormones (e.g. insulin), stimulants (e.g. ephedrine), drugs to purge fluid (e.g. diuretics), muscle growth stimulants (e.g. synthol), appetite stimulants and supplements (e.g. B12, protein powders) and syringes. In addition to the online shop, customers can access information on contests, read, and post articles on bodybuilding-related topics, and initiate or contribute to, threads in the Anabolic Steroid Discussion Forum.

Ethics

Collecting data from the Internet presents ethical challenges around what is deemed a 'public' or 'private' space. One obvious issue is whether informed consent can be gained. Some scholars (e.g. Hookway 2008) argue that open access online discussion boards, forums, and blogs are firmly located in the public domain. As such contributors

---

[2] IFBB: International Federation of Bodybuilding and Fitness, IFBB, the governing body of the sport of bodybuilding and fitness, was founded by brothers Joe and Ben Weider in 1946 in Montreal, Canada. IFBB headquarters are located in Madrid, Spain (http://www.ifbb.com/).

[3] A substance intended to enhance physical performance, stamina, or recovery.

are aware that their posts will be read by others unless they place them on a 'friends only' setting. Thus, accessible electronic talk may be "personal" but it is not "private" (Hookway 2008, p. 16) and so consent can be "waived". However, given the potentially sensitive nature of our data we deemed it appropriate to seek university ethical approval, and in line with BPS guidelines (BPS 2013), we have anonymized our dataset as far as possible (e.g. replacing tags and pseudonyms with R1 [Respondent 1], R2 etc. removing any in-text personal details or references).

Data Analysis

In analyzing our data we draw upon discourse analysis (Potter 1996). Having downloaded all 119 posts from the 17 contributors we read through our data identifying main themes (e.g. techniques, health, legality). The responses were examined further by systematic line-by-line coding. In doing so a number of sub-themes were identified (e.g. techniques: use/appearance/pain, health: cycles/safety/timing), which we contrasted and refined with others ('constant comparison' process). In addition, we identified the different discourses drawn upon so there was a dual focus on 'what' was being presented (content: synthol use) and 'how' it was being presented (process: synthol as relatively safe).

Discourse analysis, broadly speaking, helps to identify and explore how people work up versions of the world during conversational interaction (Potter 1996, p. 146). It focusses on participants' discursive practices (how discourse is used to perform specific functions) and their discursive resources (how texts are informed by wider cultural/organizational norms) (Wetherell 1998). Discourse analysis' focus on what is made relevant by participants means it avoids analyst-centred interpretations of the data. Our aim was to identify the ways in which synthol use was presented. For example, the notion that 'synthol is risky' can be analyzed with respect to the respondents' posts on drug use in sport, where distinctions are often made (e.g. uninformed user versus uniformed user) and certain groups 'othered' or denigrated in various ways (e.g. by constructing all [non]substance users as the same).

Results

Before we begin our analysis, however, we should note that all the respondents in the forum presented as men, which is not surprising since muscularity tends to be heavily associated with men and masculinity (Grogan 2008). Contributors used tags referencing traditional male names as well as positioning themselves in relation to females (e.g. the wife, Mrs.), displayed typical masculine attributes (e.g. accepting pain, constructing technical knowledge) (Young et al. 1994), and referred to each other with masculine references (e.g. brother, bro, man).

In examining the forum posts we noticed that in the absence of specialist knowledge, forum contributors worked up their authority on synthol by presenting their knowledge as credible, legitimate, and trustworthy (Epstein 1995). In particular, we noticed that some members seemed to be held in higher esteem than others; one in particular (R2). On further inspection, we ascertained that R2 was in a particularly strong position in relation to other forum contributors because he had previously published material on synthol (http://www.professional-muscle.com/forums/showthread.php?t=205). Therefore, we begin our analysis by looking at how R2's legitimation (and subsequent credibility, trust, and influence) are worked up by drawing on medical and pharmaceutical discourses as discursive resources, which serve as the basis for his unquestioned authority in the "Did My First Shots of Synthol Today!!!!" forum.

His article is too long to reproduce here in its entirety since it runs to several online pages. Therefore, we present a section of the article shortly after R2 has worked up his authority by referencing time, ubiquity, and commercial pharmaceutical legitimacy "Bristol-Myers Squibb"[4] whilst providing readers with some background.

---

[4] An American pharmaceutical company.

"Site Enhancing Oils (Synthol)— A How to Guide"

Legitimation

R2
You need to inject in EVERY head of the muscle, while rotating the shots daily within that head. This is the only way to ensure that the added size keeps to your natural look/shape of the muscle. The quickest way to get a muscle up to maximum size is to do the following regimen: 1 ml for 10 days in each head of the muscle. 2 ml for 10 days. 3 ml for 10 days. If you do both, the biceps and triceps simultaneously, you can add up to 3" on your arms in those 30 days.

How do Site Oils work? To begin with, they do not stay in the muscle for 3 to 5 years. They get dissipated within months. However, during this time, they have stretched the fascia of that muscle. The fascia is a great constrictive factor in muscle growth. The more stretched the fascia is the more the muscle will grow and the more it will have that 'popping' look. Site oils stay in there long enough for the fascia to stretch. As they dissipate, the 'space' left by them is replaced with new muscle tissue growth. That is the reason why when x-rays/MRIs were performed on some of the people that have 25" + arms, there was no oil found in there. The oil dissipated and it was replaced by real muscle .... The pain will minimise the more you inject, until it will not hurt any more. Site Oils hurt, but not as much as site injections with, let's say, Sustanon or Testosterone Propionate.

When people construct lay expertise they need to artfully anchor it to something with social credibility. Foley and Faircloth (2003) show that since medical and pharmaceutical discourses enjoy high social status, they are excellent anchoring discourses in which to build legitimacy in claims. We can see this in the way that R2 draws on medical and pharmaceutical knowledge of where to inject "in EVERY head of the muscle", appropriate dosages "1 ml for 10 days in each head of the muscle. 2 ml for 10 days. 3 ml for 10 days", the length of drug cycle "30 days", longevity of the substance in the body "They get dissipated within months", the anatomical effects "they have stretched the fascia of that muscle", its level of detection "when x-rays/MRIs were performed … no oil found" and its comparison to other pharmaceuticals "Sustanon or Testosterone Propionate". These are presented as 'facts' bolstered with claims that are presented as absolute (e.g. "This is the only way", "The quickest way") and by the use of extreme case formulations (e.g. "EVERY", "only"). Extreme case formulations are discursive devices which people draw on when describing or accounting to minimize the potential of others to refute their claims (Pomerantz 1986). We can see from the way R2 constructs his legitimacy why other forum contributors follow his advice. However, before we show how credibility from these claims is generated, maintained, and developed through the online interactions, we begin at the start of the forum thread examining the provision of support and its relation to lay expertise (Epstein 1995).

Support

Sequence 1

R1
I used 25 gauge syringes, i shot 1 cc into each bicep head, in each outer and inner bicep muscle, and the triceps also, and my problem is, my arms hurt like hell, is this normal for my muscles to hurt so bad. i messaged them real good after the injections, no lumps formed at all, i did the low weight, high reps for a warm up at the gym. Has anyone else had these muscle pains after their SYNTHOL injections. please let me know thank you

R2
Yes, that is normal. The pain will be less and less each day until after the first week you will not feel it anymore. Synthol is great stuff. You will be pleased.

R3
Yep normal. It feels a Bit like a brutal workout to where you can barely straighten your arm out all the way. In the beginning I remember many days going into work sore as can be. Just keep stretching it out and straightening your arms. As R2 said it'll get better as you go.

R4

Absolutely normal brother. Also the bruising does occur often with me, but Synthelamin B-12 calmed it a lot. But yes I did bruise most of the time. The outcome you will be impressed with so just stick with it. Keep your stock up, because with what you are doing you'll want to keep a few bottles on hand. It does go rather quickly for such a large bottle because of the large doses per day. Good luck man.

Several things stand out in this sequence. Whilst R1 opens the thread with "Did My First Shots of Synthol Today!!!!" he displays some prior knowledge of how to use synthol since he cites specific equipment ("25 gauge" syringes), dosage and location ("i shot 1 cc into each bicep head"), post-injection routine ("messaged them ... after the injections"), and subsequent gym training ("low weight, high reps for a warm up"). Although this indicates the availability of information on synthol usage, it also suggests that experiential knowledge is much scarcer: "my arms hurt like hell, is this normal for my muscles to hurt so bad". R2, 3 and 4 all provide emphatic, positive responses "Yes, that's normal", "Yep normal", "Absolutely normal brother". Studies of empathy and sympathy (Pudlinski 2005; Staske 1998) show that such responses work to normalize potentially problematic feelings and experiences by attending to them as reasonable and expectable.

R2 focuses on how long the problem will last ("after the first week you will not feel it anymore"), whilst R3 describes the pain with a training analogy ("Bit like a brutal workout") and R4 talks about the visual insults ("bruising does occur often with me"). By drawing on their own knowledge they are able to provide support for this novice; they are constructing second stories where the response is aligned to the original post (Veen et al. 2010; Sacks 1992). Second stories work to normalize group views by displaying an understanding and stance toward the initial story (Arminen 2004). What is also noticeable in these responses is that whilst the negative aspects of synthol ("lumps", "pain", "stiffness" are discussed, health risks are not; presumably because they are not known, or not acknowledged, here. What is also evident from this quote is that masculinity is also invoked in being able to tolerate pain (see Young et al. 1994 for more on pain tolerance is invoked as a normal part of sport and masculinity).

Shared experiences clearly operate to construct an event (e.g. synthol-related pain) as normative. But to move beyond empathy and support to provide advice requires positioning oneself as expert in some way.

In the next sequence we demonstrate how expertise is formulated by both the 'expert' and the 'novices'. We pick up the thread shortly a few days later after R1 posts that the pain is subsiding.

Sequence 2

Trust

R7
how the heck does one safely inject the tris? I am so afraid that I am gonna miss something because of the angle and I can't trust anyone to help me. BTW I have 25 % bf (i think) so I don't have the definition to be completely sure of where I am sticking myself.

R6
if you are at a quarter body fat, I would definitely recommend cutting down a little first. Get yourself in the 15 % range if possible otherwise you may not be able to notice the differences that Synthol makes.

R2
Agreed.
As far as injecting tris yourself:
- sit down on the floor next to the bed.
- sit at an angle, so the arm to be injected is running across the top of the bed edge
- push the arm against the bed and have the tri hanging down off the edge
- inject with the other arm, with the syringe going upwards. Very easy to inject, aspirate and push the plunger. For accuracy, look in the mirror first before you inject and mentally mark the spot.

R7
can I leave this out, or should I refrigerated it (being an oil, I would kinda doubt refrigerating it.) Also, is the plastic top self-sealing, or do I open and draw the 2CC?

R2

Room temp is fine. You draw through the top. Underneath it there's a Teflon lining which seals every time you pull the needle out.

R7

thanks for the fast response!! I will let you know how much I cry when I try tomorrow and now it also seems that I need to buy another bottle if I am to do this correctly. I got everything from the company so fast as so discretely. Well, I think discretely .... I had a sticker on both boxes saying "ID recorded" what the hell is that supposed to mean ... am I under profile?

Without the availability of online expert knowledge backed up by credentials such as academic degrees, track records, institutional affiliations and so on, trust can be an issue. R7's vulnerability display ("I am so afraid that I am gonna miss something") is reinforced by (mis-)trust issues ("I can't trust anyone to help me"). So how does he begin to trust other forum contributors that he presumably only knows online? Urban et al. (2009) point out the typical features of online trust: believable information and implied competence, confidence in the members of the online group in which members advocate other members, benevolence and integrity. We previously noted in Sequence 2 and 3 how comments from R5 and R6 positioned R2 as an expert ("you seem to be the man on this subject!"). Here we see that although R6 suggests R7's body fat is too high ("I would definitely recommend cutting down a little first") this is not responded to. Instead, R7 seems to respond instead to R2's pragmatic and technical knowledge (e.g. "… sit down on the floor next to the bed … Underneath it there's a Teflon lining which seals every time you pull the needle out"). What this shows is that R7 trusts the competence and knowledge of R2 even though R2 echoed ("Agreed") R6's suggestion of losing body fat. As Wang and Emurian (2005, p. 108) point out, one of the key elements of trust is that it is "positive". That is, actions are seen to be done for the benefit of others. Therefore, R7 can be seen to read R2's posts as honest and benevolent.

Thus far we have seen how forum members, especially R2, work up a position of trust and credibility through proving support in the form of pragmatic, health-related, and technical knowledge. In the following sequence we demonstrate how this is deployed to influence others so that they may get the best results from their synthol use whilst avoiding potential problems (e.g. lumps).

Credibility

Sequence 3

R2
Sounds good, but make sure you follow my guide, otherwise the results will not be permanent!

R5
Where can I get a list of these guidelines??? (I also need someone to use my tri's as a dartboard, but that's another story) My triceps are soooo stubborn, it's not even funny! I've beat the living piss out of them in the gym and still they are falling behind!

R2
http://www.professionalmuscle.com/forums/showthread.php?t=205

R6
R2 you seem to be the man on this subject! Help me out Bro. Is synthol just to get you over a plateau? Or can it be used just to help the growth? I know how it works (I have read your article more than a few times): D Also can you use it during your off cycle? And one more question, with 6 sticks a day in each bicep how do you prevent needle marks?: eek:

R2
You can use it for either, getting you over a plateau or to help growth. You can use it off cycle too, but ideally you should be on gear to create a maximum anabolic environment. That being said, a lot of naturals use it too. You don't do 6 injections per day in each bicep. One injection per day in each bicep head (2 injection per arm per day).

In this sequence, those seeking advice acknowledge the self-appointed expert position adopted by R2 ("Where can I get a list of these guidelines???", "you seem to be the man on this subject!"). By referencing his "guides" R2 positions himself as an authority on synthol in which being published is a social marker of status. Epstein (1995) notes that one of the defining features of credibility is the presentation of factual knowledge. This is visible in the way R2 portrays certainty: "the results will not", "You can use it for either", "you should be on gear", "You don't do 6 injections per day".

Credibility is also indexed in other ways. For example, by deploying insider community terminology (e.g. muscle talk: "getting you over a plateau or to help growth", "You can use it off cycle too") R2 displays in-group membership knowledge (Sacks 1992), which helps to provide authenticity. In addition, R2 demonstrates knowledge of two categories of bodybuilders: those who use "anabolic" steroids and those who do not, the "naturals", thus highlighting situated expertise (Mackiewicz 2010). Finally, R5 and R6's treat R2 as an expert through their questioning (e.g. "Where can I get a list of these guidelines???"), as well as in-group recognition and trust "Help me out Bro".

Having worked up legitimation, provided support and gained credibility we now focus on outcomes: trust and influence. We re-join the thread shortly after R1 has been describing how he uses heat pads to reduce any swelling in the biceps post-injection.

Sequence 4

Influence

> **R8**
> I am having a hell of a time drawing through a 25 g needle, but I have one prepped and will be prepping the second. will little bubbles be a problem? there are a few small ones, but I see they disappeared after letting the prepped needles sit for about 5 minutes.
>
> **R2**
> Draw with a 21 g and inject with a 25 g.
>
> **R8**
> it didn't even hurt. I am massaging and am out the door to hit the gym.
>
> **R8**
> ok, almost 2 hours later ... slight soreness, less than my flu shot though. feel a slight pump but no lumps. I will continue to occasionally massage the bi's

a bit through the day, especially as the soreness starts to grow (and it is now that my workout is over). gonna need to place another order for needles and synthol since 100 g will probably not be enough for a correct cycle. I have an appt on a military base hospital .... how do I hide the injection sites? I know the Docs will notice.

R2
The injections themselves don't hurt. Don't worry, the soreness will come! ;) It subsides after 1 week though. How can they notice injection sites? Needles don't leave marks unless you bruise, and then you can just say you bumped yourself. Or injected some B-12. gonna need to place another order for needles and synthol since 100 g will probably not be enough for a correct cycle. Like everything else, make sure you do it properly or you will not be happy with the results.

R8
yeah, next day I have that typical injection-in-the-muscle soreness now. one question, I can inject at work where i can close my office door, but there is no way at home on the weekends, I am rarely alone long enough and my wife would kill me if she found out. Would I suffer greatly if I skip the weekends? PS I cannot hit the Gym every day either, just not possible.

R2
First of all, you are not supposed to hit the gym every day. As far as the pumping sets after the injections, just do 2 sets of 30–50 reps with a bottle of juice in each arm, etc. You have to do the weekends. Why don't you take the syringes, etc. in the shitter and lock the door?

R8's posts describe difficulties in drawing synthol from the bottle and the related concern about "bubbles" as well as a description of post-injection soreness and detection both at work and by "Docs" at the "military base hospital". In doing so, R8 has positioned himself as a novice seeking advice from an 'expert'. R2 takes up R8's request for information by providing technical information on syringe size ("Draw with a 21 g and inject with a 25 g"), pharmaceutical quantities ("100 g will probably not be enough for a correct cycle") and duration of side effects ("soreness ... subsides after 1 week"). In doing so R2 is playing an active role in recommending correct synthol usage.

R2 also provides practical information on avoiding detection ("you bruise … just say you bumped yourself. Or injected some B-12" "Why don't you take the syringes, etc. in the shitter and lock the door") and training ("you are not supposed to hit the gym every day … do 2 sets of 30–50 reps with a bottle of juice in each arm"). Similarly to technical information, practical 'how to' information also works by highlighting the indirect benefit to the user—in this case avoiding detection (Subramani and Rajagopalan 2002). Experiential information is also provided "The injections themselves don't hurt … the soreness will come!" "make sure you do it properly or you will not be happy with the results". That is, not necessarily personal experience but information on what the recipient is likely to experience. Like the previous two examples, this type of information is presented as for the recipient's benefit. That is, if you follow my advice on a correct synthol cycle then you will "be happy with the results". Similarly to Sequence 1, by drawing on his own experience and knowledge R2 provides support and so constructs a second story (Veen et al. 2010). That is, the alignment of a second response to the original response (Sacks 1992). Whilst second stories work to normalize views displaying an understanding and stance toward the initial story they also work to add credibility to who constructs the second story (Arminen 2004). Much like a team manager may gain additional support from the team if he is drawing from personal experience rather than from learned knowledge. Therefore, what these forms of information provision demonstrate in the context of advice giving and receiving in the forum is a spreading of the word on how to use synthol and get good results whilst minimizing unwanted side effects.

Discussion

Here we have focussed on how lay expertise is worked up by Internet forum contributors when providing each other with support and advice on synthol use, to try to answer the question of how forum contributors are taken seriously. Discourse analysis of posts has shown that Epstein's (1995) five key elements of legitimation, support, credibility, trust, and influence were all evidenced in accounts. R2 used high status medical and pharmaceutical discourses, anchoring his practical knowledge and building legitimacy (Foley and Faircloth 2003). Participants R2, R3, and R4 all provided empathic, positive responses in response to reports of pain. Normalizing problematic experiences (Pudlinski 2005), and drawing on male-appropriate discourses around toughness and tolerance for pain (Young et al. 1994), operated to provide support while avoiding recognizing potential health dangers of synthol use. Expertise was formulated through implied competence. Forum members such as R2 worked up a position of credibility through focusing on pragmatic, technical knowledge, and were able to create a position of trust with others on the forum, presenting as expert users who could be trusted to provide helpful advice. Subramani and Rajagopalan's (2002) four key ways that people influence each other in social networks (benefit signalling, recommendation, signalling use, and spreading the word) were all evidence in accounts, and those seeking advice acknowledged the credibility of R2 who presented his experiences as factual, enhancing his credibility among the group (Mackiewicz 2010), and using insider terminology to provide authenticity.

Collecting our data directly from a unique forum thread where bodybuilders discussed their use of synthol enabled us to access accounts from 17 self-identified bodybuilders and to look at how they interacted with each other online when discussing, and asking for information on use This has given us some insight into a relatively new community of users without requiring them to agree to be interviewed, which may have changed and restricted what they felt able to share with a group of university academics. Obviously data are not intended to be generalized outside this group of users, though accounts have provided interesting new insights into how these users positioned themselves as novices and experts in this discussion group.

This work has important implications for promoting health in bodybuilders and others who may seek to gain the appearance of trained muscle. Although people outside the user-group may see radical differences between the cosmetically enhanced muscles created by synthol and those produced through weight training alone, seeing them as "freakish" and "bizarre" (Childs 2007), users clearly expect that synthol will give them a natural, trained look and are hungry for advice on how to use synthol and get good results whilst minimizing unwanted side effects such as pain and unsightly bumps. In the context of limited information, people with practical experience of use (such as R2) are treated with respect and trusted to provide technical and medical information which is factual and generalizable beyond personal experience of use. Clearly there is a need for medically accurate information that has credibility with bodybuilders to enable 'novice' users to have somewhere to go to find accurate information on health risks and safer use. This information needs to recognize reasons for use, and be represented using language that has credibility among the bodybuilding community.

References

Amazon.com. (2014). *Synthol posing oil—Pump and pose 100mil—3 bottles: Customer reviews*. Retrieved August 30, from http://www.amazon.com/Synthol-posing-oil-100mil-bottles/product reviews/B00B0F3FAG/ref=cm_cr_dp_qt_hist _five?ie=UTF8&filter By=addFiveStar&showViewpoints=0#reviews-container?sortBy=helpful&reviewerType=all_reviews&formatType=null&filterByStar=one_star

Arminen, I. (2004). Second stories. The saliency of interpersonal communication for mutual help in Alcoholics Anonymous. *Journal of Pragmatics, 36*, 319–347.

Arnold, M. (2014). Anabolic steroid site injections. *IronMag*. February 10. Retrieved August 30, from http://www.ironmagazine.com/2014/anabolic-steroid-site-injections/

Banke, I. J., Prodinger, P. M., Waldt, S., Weirich, G., Holzaofel, B. M., Gradinger, R., et al. (2012). Irreversible muscle damage in bodybuilding due to long-term intramuscular oil injection. *International Journal of Sports Medicine, 33*, 829–834.

Brainium, J. (2013). Inject to grow. *Iron Man Magazine*. Retrieved July 1, 2014, from http://www.ironmanmagazine.com/inject-to-grow/

British Psychological Society. (2013). Guidelines for Internet-mediated Research. Retrieved December 13, 2013, from http://www.bps.org.uk/system/files/Public%20files/inf206-guidelines-for-internet-mediated-research.pdf

Childs, D. (2007). Like implants for the arms: Synthol lures bodybuilders. *ABC News*. Retrieved June 14, 2014, from http://abcnews.go.com/Health/Fitness/story?id=3179969

Darsow, U., Bruckbauer, H., Worret, W.-I., Hofmann, H., & Ring, J. (2000). Subcutaneous oleomas induced by self-injection of sesame seed oil for muscle augmentation. *Journal of the American Academy of Dermatology, 42*, 292–294.

Di Benedetto, G., Pierangeli, M., Scalise, A., & Bertani, A. (2002). Paraffin oil injection in the body: An obsolete and destructive procedure. *Annals of Plastic Surgery, 49*, 391–396.

Epstein, S. (1995). Expertise: AIDS activism and the forging of credibility in the reform of clinical trials. *Science Technology Human Values, 20*(4), 408–437.

Foley, L., & Faircloth, C. A. (2003). Medicine as discursive resource: Legitimation in the work narratives of midwives. *Sociology of Health & Illness, 25*, 165–184.

Ghandourah, S., Hofer, M. J., Kiebling, A., El-Zayat, B., & Dietmar Schofar, M. (2012). Painful muscle fibrosis following synthol injections in a bodybuilder: A case report. *Journal of Medical Case Reports, 6*, 248.

Grogan, S. (2008). *Body image: Understanding body dissatisfaction in men, women, and children*. London: Routledge.

Hookway, N. (2008). Entering the blogosphere. Some strategies for using blogs in social research. *Qualitative Research* (8), 91.

Mackiewicz, J. (2010). The co-construction of credibility in online product reviews. *Technical Communication Quarterly, 19*(4), 403–426.

Pomerantz, A. (1986). Extreme case formulations: A way of legitimizing claims. *Human Studies, 9*, 219–229.

Potter, J. (1996). *Representing reality: Discourse, rhetoric and social construction*. London: Sage.

Pudlinski, C. (2005). Doing empathy and sympathy. Caring responses to troubles tellings on a peer support line. *Discourse Studies, 7*(3), 267–288.

Richardson, K. (2003). Health risks on the Internet: Establishing credibility on line. *Health, Risk, & Society, 5*, 171–184.

Sacks, H. (1992). In G. Jefferson (Ed.), *Lectures on conversation*. Oxford: Blackwell Publishing.

Staske, S. (1998). The normalization of problematic emotion in conversations between close relational partners. Interpersonal partner work. *Symbolic Interaction, 21*, 59–86.

Subramani, M. R., & Rajagopalan, B. (2002). *Examining viral marketing—A framework for knowledge sharing and influence in online social networks.* Management Information Systems Research Center, Working Paper # 02-12. Retrieved September 11, 2014, from http://misrc.umn.edu/workingpapers/fullPapers/2002/0212_050102.pdf

Urban, G. L., Amyxb, C., & Lorenzonc, A. (2009). Online trust: State of the art, new frontiers, and research potential. *Journal of Interactive Marketing, 23*, 179–190.

Veen, M., te Molder, H., Gremmen, B., & van Woerkum, C. (2010). Quitting is not an option. An analysis of online diet talk between celiac disease patients. *Health, 14*(1), 23–40.

Wang, Y. D., & Emurian, H. H. (2005). An overview of online trust: Concepts, elements, and implications. *Computers in Human Behavior, 21*, 105–125.

Wetherell, M. (1998). Positioning and interpretative repertoires: Conversation analysis and post-structuralism in dialogue. *Discourse & Society, 9*, 387–412.

Young, K., McTeer, W., & White, P. (1994). Body talk: Male athletes reflect on sport, injury, and pain. *Sociology of Sport Journal, 11*(2), 175–194.

Part III

Prescription Substances

9

Non-Medical Use of ADHD Stimulants for Appetite Suppression and Weight Loss

Amy J. Jeffers and Eric G. Benotsch

Non-Medical Use of Prescription Drugs

In recent years, there has been a dramatic increase in the non-medical use of prescription drugs (NMUPD), the use of psychotropic or analgesic medications (e.g. pain relievers, tranquilizers, sedatives, stimulants) without a physician's prescription, as well as the intentional misuse of one's own medication among young adults and adolescents. Consistent with the definition used in the Substance Abuse and Mental Health Services Administration's (SAMHSA) National Survey on Drug Use and Health, "NMUPD" will be used in this chapter as the umbrella term to describe use without a prescription of the individual's own, as well as intentional misuse of the individual's own prescription (e.g. intentionally using too much, using to get high, or using to enhance the effects of alcohol or other drugs; SAMHSA 2014). Thus, this is a commonly used definition that

---

A.J. Jeffers (✉), E.G. Benotsch
Virginia Commonwealth University, Department of Psychology, P.O. Box 842018, Richmond, VA 23284, United States

includes both: those who use prescription drugs without a doctor's prescription and those who intentionally misuse their own prescription drugs.

Motives for NMUPD include use to get high, for experimentation, to enhance energy, to relieve pain, and to lose weight (Jeffers et al. 2013; Jeffers and Benotsch 2014; McCabe and Cranford 2012). In national studies, as many as 29.2 % of young adults, ages 18–25, and 11.4 % of adolescents report lifetime NMUPD (Institute for Behavior and Health n.d), with almost 5 % and 2.2 % reporting NMUPD in the past month, respectively (SAMHSA 2014). In 2013, young adults and adolescents in the USA were more likely to use a prescription drug non-medically than to use any illicit substance except marijuana (SAMHSA 2014). NMUPD now accounts for more emergency room (ER) visits than the use of all illicit substances combined (SAMHSA 2012). Data from other national samples have demonstrated that NMUPD is a risk factor for future drug dependence (Schepis and Krishnan-Sarin 2008), binge drinking (McCauley et al. 2011), and substance use disorders (Schepis and Hakes 2011). NMUPD has been associated with poor mental health, including depressive symptoms, suicidality, and anxiety (Dussault and Weyandt 2013; Zullig and Divin 2012). NMUPD has also been related to sexual risk behaviour, including having more sexual partners and unprotected sex (Benotsch et al. 2011).

Non-Medical Use of Prescription Stimulants

One particularly concerning trend is the rise in the non-medical use of prescription stimulants (NMUPS; Arria and DuPont 2010; Rabiner et al. 2009). The National Survey on Drug Use and Health indicates that 603,000 people aged 12 years or older initiated NMUPS in the past year (SAMHSA 2014). Lifetime prevalence rates are estimated as high as 34 % among college students (DeSantis et al. 2008). Motivations for NMUPS include: to help with concentration, to increase alertness, to get high, and for the sake of experimenting (McCabe and Cranford 2012; Teter et al. 2006). NMUPS is associated with adverse health effects including increases in heart rate, blood pressure, body temperature, and malnutrition due to a decrease in appetite (National Institute on Drug Abuse

[NIDA] 2009). Chronic stimulant use can lead to paranoia and hostility and high doses can lead to cardiovascular consequences (NIDA 2009). Mixing prescription stimulants with drugs or alcohol can exacerbate these side effects (Higher Education Center 2012). NMUPS has been associated with the use of other substances including alcohol, tobacco, marijuana, cocaine, and ecstasy (Lanier and Farley 2011). Indeed, NMUPS has been associated with past year alcohol or drug use disorders in both adolescents and young adult men and women (Wu et al. 2007). Further, between 2005 and 2010, the number of ER visits related to NMUPS increased dramatically from 5212 to 15,585 (SAMHSA 2013). One timely concern regarding NMUPS, especially among adolescents and young adults, is their role in appetite suppression.

Pharmacology of ADHD Medications

Prescription stimulant medications used to treat ADHD, for example, Adderall and Ritalin, have shown promise for improving the main symptoms of ADHD and increasing academic performance among those with ADHD (Zachor et al. 2006). However, a common side effect of these medications is appetite suppression (Zachor et al. 2006) and subsequent weight loss (Kent et al. 1995).

There are four primary, FDA-approved, stimulant-class drugs used to treat ADHD: methylphenidate, dextroamphetamine, amphetamine, and lisdexamfetamine (Advokat et al. 2014). Each of these drugs is a sympathomimetic amine that functions as a central nervous system stimulant as well as a dopamine and norepinephrine agonist. The exact mechanism by which these stimulants improve the symptoms of ADHD is a subject of debate, but they appear to improve the functioning of the prefrontal cortex (a brain structure involved in selective attention and goal-directed behaviour) by blocking the reuptake of dopamine and norepinephrine into the presynaptic neuron, thereby increasing the availability of dopamine and norepinephrine (Advokat et al. 2014; Mariotti et al. 2013; Pliszka et al. 1996). Dextramphetamine, amphetamine, and lisdexamfetamine (but not methylphenidate) also facilitate release of dopamine and norepinephrine (Hodgkins et al. 2012). In addition, these drugs serve as dopamine agonists in the *nucleus acumbens* (a brain structure involved in pleasure) which may account for their addictive potential (Advokat et al. 2014). The appetite-suppressing effects of these medications are attributed to increased dopamine and norepinephrine activity in the hypothalamus which in turn inhibits the activity of hypothalamic neuropeptide Y (a neurotransmitter involved in appetite stimulation) (Hsieh et al. 2006; Lemieux et al. 2015).

Methylphenidate, marketed under a variety of names including Ritalin, Focalin, and Concerta is available in both immediate release and extended release oral formulations as well as an extended release dermal patch (Advokat et al. 2014). The immediate release formulations reach peak concentration in 1–2 hours and have a duration of effect of around 4 hours (Mariotti et al. 2013). Extended release formulations have a duration of effect from 7 to 12 hours, enabling individuals to take the medication only once per day (Advokat et al. 2014).

Dextroamphetamine, marketed under the names Dexedrine and Dextrostat, as well as one of the components of mixed amphetamine salt combinations (see below), is available in both immediate release and extended release oral formulations. The immediate release formulations reach peak concentrations in around 3 hours and have a duration of effect of up to 8 hours (Advokat et al. 2014). Extended release formulations have a duration of effect of up to 11 hours (Hodgkins et al. 2012).

Amphetamine (amphetamine aspartate, amphetamine sulphate) in combination with dextroamphetamine (typically described as "mixed amphetamine salts"), combined in a 1:1 ratio is marketed under the name Adderall (Advokat et al. 2014; Hodgkins et al. 2012). This medication is available in both immediate and extended release formulations. The immediate release formulation reaches peak concentration in 3 hours and has a duration of effect of 4–6 hours (Hodgkins et al. 2012). The extended release formulation has a duration of effect of up to 10 hours (Advokat et al. 2014).

The newest drug, lisdexamfetamine, is a dextroamphetamine prodrug, created by linking the amino acid lysine to dextroamphetamine (Hodgkins et al. 2012). After ingestion, the drug is then metabolized into dextroamphetamine after the lysine is cleaved during the digestion process (Advokat et al. 2014). The intent with this formulation was to reduce the drug's abuse potential, as crushing and then injecting the drug or crushing for intranasal consumption does not lead to rapid euphoric effects (Hodgkins et al. 2012). Lisdexamfetamine is marketed under the name Vyvanse. Because it has to be metabolized in order to be activated, it is available as an extended release formulation only. It reaches peak concentration in 3.5 hours and has a duration of effect of up to 14 hours (Hodgkins et al. 2012).

Off-Label Use of ADHD Medications for Weight Loss

It has been well understood for some time that the stimulant drugs used to treat ADHD have appetite-suppressing and subsequent weight loss effects, especially during the first 6 months of use (Lisska and Rivkees 2003). Indeed, children who are prescribed stimulant ADHD medications grow more slowly than their non-medicated peers (Poulton 2005). Recent work suggests that the anorexic effects of these stimulants also affect body composition, including reductions in both adipose and lean body tissue as well as reduced bone mineral density (Poulton et al. 2012). In a prospective cohort study of Italian children, Ruggiero et al. (2012) found that weight loss was the most commonly reported adverse reaction among children prescribed stimulant medications for ADHD. Some work suggests that use of mixed dextroamphetamine-amphetamine salts (Adderall) results in greater weight loss (or more attenuated weight gain) than use of methylphenidate (Pliszka et al. 2006).

In a novel test of the potential of ADHD medications to promote weight loss, Levy et al. (2009) screened severely obese patients for ADHD and identified 78 individuals who met criteria for the diagnosis. These individuals were prescribed ADHD medications, primarily stimulant medications, although 9 % of the enrolled participants received only a non-stimulant ADHD medication (atomoxetine). Participants who could not tolerate the medications (n = 13, 17 %) served as controls. All participants were also offered dietary counselling. These individuals were followed for an average of 15 months. Compared to control participants, who gained an average of 3.26 kg (> 2 % of initial body weight) in the follow-up period, medicated participants lost an average of 15.05 kg (> 12 % of initial body weight), a statistically significant difference.

Currently, the only stimulant medication used to treat ADHD that has FDA-approval for a weight-related condition is lisdexamfetamine (Vyvanse), which is approved for the treatment of moderate to severe binge eating disorder (Citrome 2015). Randomized controlled trials suggest that lisdexamfetamine is effective in reducing the frequency of binge eating episodes (Citrome 2015; McElroy et al. 2015). Although these trials also documented weight loss averaging 5–7 % of initial weight, the FDA has not approved this medication for the treatment of obesity (Citrome 2015).

Although stimulant ADHD medications are not currently FDA-approved for weight loss, media reports suggest that some physicians prescribe them "off-label" for this purpose, typically in individuals who are obese and for whom other treatments have not been effective (Bernstein 2006; Johnson 2006). Prescribing a medication for a purpose other than one for which it has received FDA-approval ("off-label"—meaning that specified use is not listed on the FDA-required drug label provided by the manufacturer) is legal in the USA provided that the health-care provider can articulate some rationale for the off-label use (Trenque et al. 2014). Some research suggests that off-label prescriptions for methylphenidate are associated with a greater likelihood of adverse reactions (Trenque et al. 2014). That study assessed off-label use when the medication was prescribed by a physician. Of course, individuals who are self-administering ADHD prescription stimulants for weight loss without the advice of a physician are also engaged in off-label use, and given the lack of involvement of a medical professional, may be at higher risk for adverse reactions.

Despite the media attention, relatively little systematic research has been conducted examining physician prescribing of ADHD stimulant medications off-label for the purpose of weight loss. In the one study that has examined this topic, Brinker et al. (2007) used prescription claims data from a large, U.S.-based national database to determine the physician-identified purpose for prescribing an ADHD medication. Prescriptions written for 43,175 unique patients were examined and the associated disease codes were almost exclusively for a psychiatric diagnosis (typically ADHD, with smaller numbers for narcolepsy and depression), and not for the treatment of obesity or for the purpose of weight loss. It should be noted that the records examined were for 2004. It is unknown if off-label use of ADHD stimulants for weight loss has increased since that time, but this is an area ripe for future research.

NMUPS for Weight Loss

Because of the widely known appetite-suppressing and weight loss effects of ADHD medications, and given the increasing number of young adults and adolescents who are dissatisfied with their bodies (Bucchianeri et al. 2013) and report a desire to lose weight (Neumark-Sztainer et al. 2011), some individuals are motivated to misuse these drugs for the purpose of losing weight (Jeffers et al. 2013; Jeffers and Benotsch 2014). Further, there is a wide misperception that prescription drugs are safe even when taken without a prescription (NIDA 2013). This misperception and the ease of obtaining these substances contribute to their frequent non-medical use. Indeed, many individuals who share medications are unaware of their dangers and procure them for free from a friend or relative (NIDA 2013). Thus, stimulant medication may seem like an inexpensive, easy way to lose weight. Engaging in the non-medical use of prescription ADHD medication for the purpose of weight loss/appetite suppression has been discussed in the popular press, and is beginning to gain attention in scientific literature (e.g. DeSantis et al. 2008; Jeffers et al. 2013; Jeffers and Benotsch 2014; Rabiner et al. 2009; Teter et al. 2006).

While this body of literature is growing, few studies discuss this phenomenon as the focal point of the research. In one study, the non-medical use of specific prescription stimulants was examined along with the motives for such use in a random sample of college students attending a single university (Teter et al. 2006). About 9.7 % ($n = 37$) of the lifetime users reported using stimulants not prescribed to them for the purpose of weight loss. However, this motivation was the sixth highest reason given after motives such as improving concentration, use as a study aid, and increasing alertness; thus, the use of prescription stimulants for weight loss was minimally examined in this study. Rabiner et al. (2009) examined the misuse of ADHD medication among individuals who reported having a current prescription for these medications ($N = 115$), of which 27 (23.5 %) reported misuse. Motivations for misusing prescription stimulants were discussed, including for the purpose of losing weight. However, this was not a focus of the research as this behaviour was minimally endorsed within the sample. Judson and Langdon (2009) found that 3.6 % of individuals reported non-medically using ADHD medication to lose weight in a sample of 333 students (both prescription and non-prescription holders). McCabe and Cranford (2012) examined motivations for NMUPD in a nationally representative sample of high school seniors. Approximately 11.3 % (n = 1399) of the entire sample reported non-medical use of at least one prescription medication in the past year. Prescription stimulants were the largest class of non-medically used drugs (7.2 %). Motivations for individuals who engaged in NMUPD included to increase energy (56.8 %), to experiment (54.6 %), to stay awake (47.7 %), and to help with weight loss (35.5 %).

NMUPS for Weight Loss as a Focal Point

Although the previous studies mention weight loss as a motivation of NMUPS, only a few studies discuss this phenomenon at length; however, these studies were investigating stimulant misuse in general. In a literature review on NMUPS among college students, Flory et al. (2014) found that the most commonly endorsed motives were academic-related. However, as McCabe and Cranford (2012) point out, most individuals have more than one motive for engaging in NMUPD, and understanding more about these motivations is vital for the development of appropriate prevention and intervention programs. Further, because society is increasingly focussed on physical appearance, with emphasis on the thin-ideal for women and muscularity for men (Leit et al. 2001; Mazur 1986), adolescents and young adults may seek out novel ways to lose weight in an attempt to attain this ideal standard. Thus, as is evident from the previously mentioned studies, NMUPS for weight loss is appealing to some individuals and the topic has gained increasing attention. In 2008, DeSantis and colleagues examined the non-medical use of prescription ADHD medications among college students and found that among the 585 participants that reported use without a prescription, 5 % reported using for the purpose of suppressing appetite. This motive was also mentioned in qualitative interviews the researchers conducted. For some participants, appetite suppression was a beneficial side effect to use, and for some it was the primary motive. For example, one participant who reported studying as the main motive of NMUPS said, "It is kind of cool that you also don't want to eat either" (DeSantis et al. 2008). Other participants discussed engaging in NMUPS for weight loss, especially for special occasions, including spring break and fraternity formal gatherings. One woman reported, "Sometimes you need a little help. You put on a little weight, and you know you have to get in a tight dress. It really takes your hunger away for a few days. I don't use it all the time though, no. But sometimes, you have no choice" (DeSantis et al. 2008).

To our knowledge, there are only two studies to date that have focussed specifically on NMUPS for the purpose of weight loss (Jeffers et al. 2013; Jeffers and Benotsch 2014). In 2013, we found that 11.7 % of young adults ($N = 705$) surveyed reported having used a prescription stimulant for the purpose of losing weight. Use was comparable across genders, age, and body mass index (BMI) between participants who utilized prescription stimulants for weight loss and non-users. However, White participants were more likely to report engaging in the behaviour than non-White participants.

Individuals who reported using prescription stimulants for weight loss were more likely to report dieting, had lower self-esteem, and had greater appearance-related motivations for weight loss (e.g. to be more accepted by society and to be better liked) compared to health-oriented motivations (e.g. to decrease their health risks and live longer). We also investigated constructs regarding stress-eating (i.e. eating as a coping mechanism that occurs in response to a particular emotion or stressor), as well as appraisal of stressors, which involved examining individuals' perceptions of their abilities to change a situation; control emotional reactions; and effectively cope. We found that prescription stimulant users had a more compromised appraisal of their ability to cope (e.g. not capable of dealing with stressful situations), and they also had greater emotion and stress-related eating (e.g. overeat when stressed). Finally, prescription stimulant users were more likely to report engaging in other unhealthy weight loss and eating disordered behaviours such as vomiting, using laxatives, utilizing a fad diet, smoking cigarettes for weight loss, and skipping meals. Indeed, individuals were eight times more likely to engage in these behaviours.

While this study provided additional evidence that a substantial minority of college students are engaging in this behaviour, we did not clearly differentiate between those who misused their own ADHD medication for the purpose of weight loss (i.e. for a purpose other than was intended) from those who received medication from another source (i.e. non-medical use).

We also conducted follow-up work that examined young adults ($N = 707$) NMUPS, in general and for weight loss, other recreational and illicit drug use, perceived effectiveness of NMUPS for weight loss, eating disordered behaviours and symptomatology, and body image (Jeffers and Benotsch 2014). Current ADHD prescription holders were excluded in this study given that these medications are sometimes prescribed off-label for weight loss (Bernstein 2006), and we wanted to account for this possibility. Moreover, we wanted to focus the investigation on users who did not actually have a prescription but were getting the medication from another source, as these individuals are typically at great risk for adverse effects (e.g. cardiac effects; Benson et al. 2015). Approximately 4.4 % of the sample engaged in NMUPS for weight loss. This rate is lower than that found in our prior study, however, the exclusion of prescription holders might account for some of the variability. As with the last study, NMUPS for weight loss was comparable across genders and was unrelated to age. However, there were significant differences in BMI between participants reporting the behaviour and those who did not, such that the former group had a lower BMI. Also, race/ethnicity was not related to NMUPS for weight loss, unlike the previous study. Of those reporting the behaviour, more than half reported receiving the medication from friends (56.7 %), with the remaining receiving from family (13.3 %), from a stranger (10 %), and from the Internet (3.3 %), consistent with previous research (NIDA 2013). About a third (35.7 %) responded that this weight loss strategy was "mildly effective", 21.4 % "not at all effective", 21.4 % "somewhat effective", and 21.4 % "very effective".

Individuals who engaged in NMUPS for weight loss had problematic attitudes and feelings related to eating, including a high level of concern regarding dieting and weight. These individuals also engaged in problematic eating behaviours and had higher eating disorder symptomatology. Indeed, vomiting to control weight and shape as well as laxative, diet pill, or diuretic use was robustly associated with NMUPS for weight loss. There was also an association with binge eating, but this relation did not hold when examined from a multivariate perspective. There were also no differences between groups regarding excessive exercise (i.e. more than 60 minutes a day) and excessive weight loss (i.e. 20 pounds or more in the past 6 months). Individuals who engaged in NMUPS for weight loss had lower body appreciation and higher body image concerns, specifically related to the media. We used the Sociocultural Attitudes Towards Appearance Scale-3 (SATAQ-3; Thompson et al. 2004) to assess sociocultural influences on body image and eating disturbances, and found that individuals scored higher on three of the four SATAQ-3 subscales: internalization-general (i.e. internalization of overall societal appearance norms), pressures (i.e. perceived pressures from the media to achieve the sociocultural appearance ideal), and information (i.e. media as an important source of information regarding appearance). Poorer body image among these individuals is consistent with prior research in that individuals who engage in disordered eating behaviours tend to have higher body image concerns (Thompson et al. 1999). Finally, individuals were also more likely to use illicit drugs, including marijuana, cocaine, methamphetamine, and hallucinogens.

This non-medical use is especially concerning given the importance of body image and weight during young adulthood, within the college setting in particular. Indeed, the college environment has been implicated in the development of body dissatisfaction and disordered eating (Fitzsimmons-Craft 2011), and individuals may be especially prone to seek out novel ways to lose weight. Moreover, college students non-medically using ADHD medication for school-related purposes (e.g. increase concentration) may perceive the weight loss side-effect to be an added bonus, thus increasing their desire to misuse.

NMUPS for Weight Loss and Stigma

Prior research has demonstrated that the most commonly endorsed motives for NMUPS among college students are related to academics (Flory et al. 2014), but it could be that individuals are underreporting stimulant use for weight loss due to a perceived stigma surrounding misusing one's medication or engaging in non-medical use for a less "acceptable" purpose. For example, Lookatch et al. (2014) studied the impact of both gender and motivations on college students' perceptions of NMUPS using vignettes, which included either a college man or woman engaging in NMUPS for one of three motives: get high, study, or lose weight. They found that, regardless of gender, using a prescription stimulant as a study aid was viewed more favourably than for the purposes of getting high or losing weight. One explanation the authors gave for the greater acceptability of using a stimulant to study was because of the similarity to the medication's intended uses, such that individuals with ADHD are often prescribed the medication to improve concentration and attention. Thus, an individual without ADHD using the medication for the same purposes is seen as acceptable. Consequently, college students may be more willing to share their experiences with NMUPS regarding "acceptable" study motives, compared with using the medication as a weight loss aid.

NMUPS for Weight Loss and Demographic

Additionally, Lookatch et al. (2014) speculate that one reason there was no difference in the acceptability of NMUPS for weight loss across gender could be that both men and women are increasingly affected by society's emphasis on achieving the ideal body type, and are therefore more willing to engage in unhealthy ways to achieve that standard. Indeed, in both of our studies (Jeffers et al. 2013; Jeffers and Benotsch 2014), NMUPS for weight loss was comparable across genders. Like women, men are increasingly concerned about body image and weight (Pope et al. 1997) and are not immune to engaging in unhealthy weight loss behaviours (Petrie et al. 2008). DeSantis et al. (2008), however, stated that a disproportionate number of women in their study talked about using stimulants for their appetite suppressive effects, although they did not give percentages by gender.

Further, there are mixed findings regarding racial/ethnic demographics. In our 2013 study (Jeffers et al. 2013), Whites were significantly more likely to misuse stimulants for weight loss than non-Whites. However, in our 2014 study (Jeffers and Benotsch 2014), Whites and non-Whites reported similar rates of this behaviour. The former finding is consistent with research that indicates Whites are more likely to engage in NMUPD in general (Young et al. 2012) as well as disordered eating behaviours (Striegel-Moore et al. 2003). However, the racial/ethnic gap regarding weight concerns and related behaviours may be closing. Indeed, Neumark-Sztainer et al. (2002) found that among adolescents, weight-related concerns (e.g. body dissatisfaction) and behaviours (e.g. vomiting) are prevalent regardless of racial/ethnic background. Overall, more research is needed to examine who is most likely to engage in this behaviour.

Limitations of the Current Research and Future Directions

Although promising, limitations of the existing research concerning NMUPS for weight loss include the exclusive use of college student samples, scant qualitative research, and relatively little attention to relevant health behaviour theory.

NMUPS in College Students and Non-College Students

The majority of studies examining NMUPS among young adults have focussed on college students as prevalence rates of NMUPS are typically higher in this population compared to their non-college, same-age peers (Herman-Stahl et al. 2007). This is not surprising given the commonly reported motives for NMUPS related to improving academic performance (Herman-Stahl et al. 2007). College students may also have greater exposure to individuals using prescription medications (both for medical and non-medical purposes) (Herman-Stahl et al. 2007). However, NMUPS prevalence rates vary and range from 3 to 36 % (McCabe et al. 2006) in college student samples depending on geographic location and school admission standards (Gallucci 2011).

Relatively few studies have examined NMUPS in non-college populations (e.g. Herman-Stahl et al. 2007; Wu et al. 2007). While there is evidence to support higher prevalence rates in college populations, non-college young adults are also at risk for engaging in this behaviour. Kelly et al. (2013) found that in a sample of socially active young adults who participate in urban nightlife (N = 1207), 44.1 % reported lifetime NMUPD, with NMUPS as the most prevalent in the past 6 months (16.7 %). Although the authors did not report on college attendance rates, it is probable that this community sample consisted of both students and non-students. As the authors concluded, a contribution of this study included moving beyond college student samples to lend insight into non-medical use across a spectrum of young adults (Kelly et al. 2013). Additionally, results from the 2013 Monitoring the Future survey demonstrated that annual prevalence rates of Adderall use were somewhat higher for college students (9.0 %), but 6.7 % of their non-college peers also endorsed the behaviour (Johnston et al. 2013). Further, prevalence rates of Ritalin are much lower than rates of Adderall but rates were not different for college students (1.8 %) and non-college students (2.6 %).

Clearly, NMUPS is not limited to undergraduate students. Further, although most research suggests higher rates in college student populations, prevalence rates are concerning in their non-college counterparts (e.g. 6.7 %; Johnston et al. 2013). Moreover, academic-related motives for NMUPS (e.g. improve academic performance) are undoubtedly more salient among college students, but it is likely that non-academic related motives (e.g. appetite suppression) are just as prevalent among non-college populations. Research is warranted to examine NMUPS in national samples of young adults in order to gain a more comprehensive picture of the behaviour, specifically as it relates to weight loss.

Importance of Examining NMUPS for Weight Loss During Adolescence

Additionally, future work is warranted with adolescents as they are the second largest age group (following young adults) to engage in NMUPD (SAMHSA 2014). Previous studies suggest that NMUPS for weight loss is associated with problematic weight-related motivations, behaviours, and other substance use. However, to date these relations have only been examined in young adult, college students. Further, it is unclear from the current literature when these adults started engaging in NMUPS for weight loss. Only one study has examined motivations for NMUPD in a nationally representative sample of high school seniors, and, as previously mentioned, prescription stimulants were the largest class of non-medically used drugs (McCabe and Cranford 2012). Notably, 35.5 % of individuals who reported NMUPS indicated doing so to help with weight loss.

Other Substance Use and NMUPD During Adolescence

Investigation into NMUPS for weight loss in adolescents is needed, as data suggest NMUPD often begins during this developmental stage (Wilens et al. 2008; Young et al. 2012). A systematic review of NMUPD among adolescents found that illicit drug use was associated with NMUPD; thus, it is likely that such individuals are engaging in polysubstance use (Young et al. 2012). Indeed, adolescents who engage in NMUPS are more likely to use illicit drugs, such as marijuana and inhalants (Nakawaki and Crano 2012). NMUPS can begin as early as grade school (Wilens et al. 2008). A systematic review examining the misuse and diversion of medications prescribed for ADHD found that children with medications receive requests to give, sell, or trade them to other students in elementary and high school (Wilens et al. 2008). Further, adolescents with stimulant prescriptions for ADHD are more likely to be approached to divert their medications compared to individuals with prescriptions for pain, anti-anxiety, and sleeping medications (McCabe et al. 2011).

Disordered Eating and Weight Control Behaviours

Adolescence is a common time for the onset of eating disorder symptoms and unhealthy weight control behaviours (Hoste et al. 2012; Neumark-Sztainer et al. 2011; Rawana et al. 2010; Vander Wal 2012). Not only is the prevalence of disordered eating and dieting high in adolescence, but individuals who engaged in these behaviours during adolescence had a heightened risk of continuation of these behaviours ten years later (Neumark-Sztainer et al. 2011). Indeed, subthreshold forms of eating disorders in adolescence have a high likelihood of transitioning to threshold levels later in life (Neumark-Sztainer et al. 2006, 2009, 2011).

Given that body dissatisfaction is high during adolescence, youth may seek out novel weight loss methods to attain society's ideal body. Thus, it is likely that NMUPS for weight loss is appealing to some. Because most adolescents who engage in NMUPD procure the drugs for free from a friend or relative, stimulant medication may seem like a cheap, simple way to lose weight. Research is needed to further investigate NMUPS for weight loss and possible correlates in samples of adolescents from a wider age range (other than high school seniors), and more diverse ethnic/racial groups.

Additional Future Directions

Because NMUPS for weight loss is associated with poor psychosocial health and health-jeopardizing behaviours, further research is warranted to examine factors such as motivations and attitudes that are amenable to change. A limitation of these prior studies is that they were largely atheoretical. Future research may benefit from applying health behaviour theory to this problematic behaviour, as doing so may provide a useful framework for better understanding the constructs related to NMUPS for weight loss, which can aid in developing interventions.

The paucity of literature also warrants further investigation of individuals' knowledge concerning the medication including side-effects, contraindications, and risks of the medication, and how individuals are (or are not) made aware of such information (e.g. friend). Future research should also assess perceived safety, negative consequences associated with NMUPS (e.g. ER visits), age of onset, how they decided to try this behaviour, situations that promote this behaviour, and whether individuals engage in NMUPS for weight loss concurrently with other unhealthy weight loss and disordered eating behaviours. Further, future qualitative work may aid in answering some of these questions. While prior studies utilizing quantitative surveys have informed information regarding prevalence rates of NMUPS for weight loss in various samples, as well as associations with other health behaviours and psychological correlates, a finer grained picture is needed to fully understand this behaviour. Thus, qualitative research is warranted to aid in the exploration of this research and to gain a complex, detailed understanding of the issue. In particular, it is important to capture the "essence" of the behaviour by understanding experiences of NMUPS for weight loss and the context and situations that influence the behaviour. Additionally, answers that are not easily captured in quantitative surveys (or are limited in their response), such as the advantages/disadvantages to losing weight this way, and when participants started engaging in this behaviour and why would benefit from qualitative inquiry. Moreover, qualitative methodology has typically been neglected in past NMUPD research (DeSantis et al. 2008), and especially with regard to NMUPS for weight loss. Finally, it would be useful to examine the prevalence of off-label use of ADHD stimulants for weight loss and possible consequences associated with use.

Conclusions

A substantial minority of college students are obtaining prescription stimulant medication for the appetite suppression and weight loss effects. Research has demonstrated that this non-medical use is related to disordered eating behaviours; other substance use; and psychological concerns, including body dissatisfaction. While there have been mixed results regarding who engages in this behaviour, prescription stimulants may be appealing to both men and women (as well as individuals of varying race/ethnicities) as this method of weight loss may not seem as "extreme" as other methods, such as vomiting. Prospective research is needed to further examine this behaviour in other populations (e.g. non-college young adults, adolescents), utilizing various methodologies (e.g. qualitative inquiry), and relevant health behaviour theory.

Eating disorder prevention and intervention programs should consider assessing NMUPS for weight loss and educating young adults about associated dangers. Clinicians should also include this behaviour when assessing unhealthy weight loss practices. When prescribing ADHD medications, physicians should emphasize the harmful consequences associated with sharing prescriptions and taking medications for purposes other than intended. NMUPD awareness campaigns should include information regarding NMUPS for weight loss and negative health consequences.

References

Advokat, C. D., Comaty, J. E., & Julien, R. M. (2014). *Julien's primer of drug action* (13th ed.). New York: Worth.

Arria, A. M., & DuPont, R. L. (2010). Nonmedical prescription stimulant use among college students: Why we need to do something and what we need to do. *Journal of Addictive Diseases, 29*, 417–426. doi:10.1080/10550887.2010.509273.

Benotsch, E. G., Koester, S., Luckman, D., Martin, A., & Cejka, A. (2011). Non-medical use of prescription drugs and sexual risk behavior in young adults. *Addictive Behaviors, 36*, 152–155.

Benson, K., Flory, K., Humphreys, K. L., & Lee, S. S. (2015). Misuse of stimulant medication among college students: A comprehensive review and meta-analysis. *Clinical Child and Family Psychology Review, 18*, 50–76. doi:10.1007/s10567-014-0177-z.

Bernstein, E. (2006). A new breed of 'diet' pills. *Wall Street Journal.* Available at: http://www.wsj.com/articles/SB115620617571041689

Brinker, A., Mosholder, A., Schech, S. D., Burgess, M., & Avigan, M. (2007). Indication and use of drug products used to treat attention-deficit/hyperactivity disorder: A cross-sectional study with inference on the likelihood of treatment in adulthood. *Journal of Child and Adolescent Psychopharmacology, 17*, 328–333.

Bucchianeri, M. M., Arikian, A. J., Hannan, P. J., Eisenberg, M. E., & Neumark-Sztainer, D. (2013). Body dissatisfaction from adolescence to young adulthood: Findings from a 10-year longitudinal study. *Body Image, 10*(1), 1–7. doi:10.1016/j.bodyim.2012.09.001.

Citrome, L. (2015). Lisdexamfetamine for binge eating disorder in adults: A systematic review of the efficacy and safety profile for this newly approved indication—What is the number needed to treat, number needed to harm and likelihood to be helped or harmed? *International Journal of Clinical Practice, 69*, 410–421.

DeSantis, A. D., Webb, E. M., & Noar, S. M. (2008). Illicit use of prescription ADHD medications on a college campus: A multimethodological approach. *Journal of American College Health, 57*(3), 315–324. doi:10.3200/JACH.57.3.315-324.

Dussault, C. L., & Weyandt, L. L. (2013). An examination of prescription stimulant misuse and psychological variables among sorority and fraternity college populations. *Journal of Attention Disorders, 17*(2), 87–97. doi:10.1177/1087054711428740.

Fitzsimmons-Craft, E. E. (2011). Social psychological theories of disordered eating in college women: Review and integration. *Clinical Psychology Review, 31*(7), 1224–1237.

Flory, K., Payne, R. A., & Benson, K. (2014). Misuse of prescription stimulant medication among college students: Summary of the research literature and clinical recommendations. *Journal of Clinical Outcomes Management, 21*(12), 559–568.

Gallucci, A. R. (2011). *A survey examining the nonmedical use and diversion of prescription stimulant medications among college students using the Theory of Planned Behavior.* Doctoral dissertation. The University of Alabama. Retrieved from http://acumen.lib.ua.edu/content/u0015/0000001/0000552/u0015_0000001_0000552.pdf

Herman-Stahl, M. A., Krebs, C. P., Kroutil, L. A., & Heller, D. C. (2007). Risk and protective factors for methamphetamine use and nonmedical use of prescription stimulants among young adults aged 18 to 25. *Addictive Behaviors, 32*(5), 1003–1015. doi:10.1016/j.addbeh.2006.07.010.

Higher Education Center. (2012). Prescription stimulants: Ritalin, Adderall, Concerta, Dexedrine. Retrieved from http://www.higheredcenter.org/highrisk/drugs/ritalin

Hodgkins, P., Shaw, M., McCarthy, S., & Sallee, F. R. (2012). The pharmacology and clinical outcomes of amphetamines to treat ADHD. *CNS Drugs, 26*, 245–268.

Hoste, R. R., Labuschagne, Z., & Le Grange, D. (2012). Adolescent bulimia nervosa. *Current Psychiatry Reports, 14*(4), 391–397.

Hsieh, Y. S., Yang, S. F., Chiou, H. L., & Kuo, D. Y. (2006). Activations of c-*fos*/c-*jun* signaling are involved in the modulation of hypothalamic superoxide dismutate (SOD) and neuropeptide Y (NPY) gene expression in amphetamine-mediated appetite suppression. *Toxicology and Applied Pharmacology, 212*, 99–109.

Institute for Behavior and Health. (n.d). *Prescription drug abuse.* Retrieved from http://www.ibhinc.org/pda.html

Jeffers, A., Benotsch, E. G., & Koester, S. (2013). Misuse of prescription stimulants for weight loss, psychosocial variables, and eating disordered behaviors. *Appetite, 65*, 8–13. doi:10.1016/j.appet.2013.01.008.

Jeffers, A. J., & Benotsch, E. G. (2014). Non-medical use of prescription stimulants for weight loss, disordered eating, and body image. *Eating Behaviors, 15*(3), 414–418. doi:10.1016/j.eatbeh.2014.04.019.

Johnson, C. (2006). Off-label drugs prescribed for weight loss. *CBS News*. Available at: http://www.cbsnews.com/news/off-label-drugs-prescribed-for-weight-loss/

Johnston, L. D., O'Malley, P. M., Bachman, J. G., & Schulenberg, J. E. (2013). *Monitoring the future national survey results on drug use, 1975–2012: Volume 2, College students and adults ages 19–50*. Ann Arbor: Institute for Social Research, The University of Michigan.

Judson, R., & Langdon, S. W. (2009). Illicit use of prescription stimulants among college students: Prescription status, motives, theory of planned behaviour, knowledge and self-diagnostic tendencies. *Psychology, Health & Medicine, 14*(1), 97–104. doi:10.1080/13548500802126723.

Kelly, B. C., Wells, B. E., Leclair, A., Tracy, D., Parsons, J. T., & Golub, S. A. (2013). Prevalence and correlates of prescription drug misuse among socially active young adults. *International Journal of Drug Policy, 24*(4), 297–303. doi:10.1016/j.drugpo.2012.09.002.

Kent, J. D., Blader, J. C., Koplewicz, H. S., Abikoff, H., & Foley, C. A. (1995). Effects of late-afternoon methylphenidate administration on behavior and sleep in attention-deficit hyperactivity disorder. *Pediatrics, 96*(2), 320–325.

Lanier, C., & Farley, E. J. (2011). What matters most? Assessing the influence of demographic characteristics, college-specific risk factors, and poly-drug use on nonmedical prescription drug use. *Journal of American College Health, 59*(8), 721–727. doi:10.1080/07448481.2010.546463.

Leit, R. A., Pope, H. G., & Gray, J. J. (2001). Cultural expectations of muscularity in men: The evolution of Playgirl centerfolds. *International Journal of Eating Disorders, 29*, 90–93.

Lemieux, A. M., Li, B., & al'Absi, M. (2015). Khat use and appetite: An overview and comparison of amphetamine, khat, and cathinone. *Journal of Ethnopharmacology, 160*, 78–85.

Levy, L. D., Fleming, J. P., & Klar, D. (2009). Treatment of refractory obesity in severely obese adults following management of newly diagnosed attention deficit hyperactivity disorder. *International Journal of Obesity, 33*, 326–334.

Lisska, M. C., & Rivkees, S. A. (2003). Daily methylphenidate use slows the growth of children: A community based study. *Journal of Pediatric Endocrinology & Metabolism, 16*, 711–718.

Lookatch, S. J., Moore, T. M., & Katz, E. C. (2014). Effects of gender and motivations on perceptions of nonmedical use of prescription stimulants. *Journal of American College Health, 62*(4), 255–262. doi:10.1080/07448481.2014.891593.

Mariotti, K. C., Rossato, L. G., Fröehlich, P. E., & Limberger, R. P. (2013). Amphetamine-type medicines: A review of pharmacokinetics, pharmacodynamics, and toxicological aspects. *Current Clinical Pharmacology, 8*, 350–357.

Mazur, A. (1986). U.S. trends in feminine beauty and overadaptation. *Journal of Sex Research, 22*, 281–303.

McCabe, S. E., & Cranford, J. A. (2012). Motivational subtypes of nonmedical use of prescription medications: Results from a national study. *Journal of Adolescent Health, 51*(5), 445–452. doi:10.1016/j.jadohealth.2012.02.004.

McCabe, S. E., Teter, C. J., & Boyd, C. J. (2006). Medical use, illicit use and diversion of prescription stimulant medication. *Journal of Psychoactive Drugs, 38*(1), 43–56.

McCabe, S. E., West, B. T., Teter, C. J., Ross-Durow, P., Young, A., & Boyd, C. J. (2011). Characteristics associated with the diversion of controlled medications among adolescents. *Drug and Alcohol Dependence, 118*(2–3), 452–458.

McCauley, J. L., Amstadter, A. B., Macdonald, A., Kmett Danielson, C., Ruggiero, K. J., Resnick, H. S., et al. (2011). Non-medical use of prescription drugs in a national sample of college women. *Addictive Behaviors, 36*, 690–695.

McElroy, S. L., Hudson, J. I., Mitchell, J. E., Wilfley, D., Ferreira-Cornwell, M. C., Gao, J., et al. (2015). Efficacy and safety of lisdexamfetamine for treatment of adults with moderate to severe binge-eating disorder. *JAMA Psychiatry, 72*, 235–246.

Nakawaki, B., & Crano, W. D. (2012). Predicting adolescents' persistence, nonpersistence, and recent onset of nonmedical use of opioids and stimulants. *Addictive Behaviors, 37*(6), 716–721.

National Institute on Drug Abuse. (2009). *DrugFacts: Stimulant ADHD medications—Methylphenidate and amphetamines.* Retrieved from http://www.drugabuse.gov/publications/drugfacts/stimulant-adhd-medications-methylphenidate-amphetamines

National Institute on Drug Abuse. (2013). *DrugFacts: Prescription and over-the-counter medications*. Retrieved from http://www.drugabuse.gov/publications/drugfacts/prescription-over-counter-medications

Neumark-Sztainer, D., Croll, J., Story, M., Hannan, P. J., French, S. A., & Perry, C. (2002). Ethnic/racial differences in weight-related concerns and behaviors among adolescent girls and boys: Findings from project EAT. *Journal of Psychosomatic Research, 53*, 963–974.

Neumark-Sztainer, D., Wall, M., Guo, J., Story, M., Haines, J., & Eisenberg, M. (2006). Obesity, disordered eating, and eating disorders in a longitudinal study of adolescents: How do dieters fare 5 years later? *Journal of the American Dietetic Association, 106*, 559–568.

Neumark-Sztainer, D., Wall, M., Larson, N. I., Eisenberg, M. E., & Loth, K. (2011). Dieting and disordered eating behaviors from adolescence to young adulthood: Findings from a 10-year longitudinal study. *Journal of the American Dietetic Association, 111*(7), 1004–1011. doi:10.1016/j.jada.2011.04.012.

Neumark-Sztainer, D., Wall, M., Story, M., & Sherwood, N. E. (2009). Five-year longitudinal predictive factors for disordered eating in a population-based sample of overweight adolescents: Implications for prevention and treatment. *International Journal of Eating Disorders, 42*, 664–672.

Petrie, T. A., Greenleaf, C., Reel, J., & Carter, J. (2008). Prevalence of eating disorders and disordered eating behaviors among male collegiate athletes. *Psychology of Men & Masculinity, 9*(4), 267–277.

Pliszka, S. R., Matthews, T. L., Braslow, K. J., & Watson, M. A. (2006). Comparative effects of methylphenidate and mixed salts amphetamine on height and weight in children with attention-deficit/hyperactivity disorder. *Journal of the American Academy of Child and Adolescent Psychiatry, 45*, 520–526.

Pliszka, S. R., McCracken, J. T., & Maas, J. W. (1996). Catecholamines in attention-deficit hyperactivity disorder: Current perspectives. *Journal of the American Academy of Child and Adolescent Psychiatry, 35*, 264–272.

Pope, H. G., Gruber, A. J., Choi, P., Olivardia, R., & Phillips, K. A. (1997). Muscle dysmorphia: An underrecognized form of body dysmorphic disorder. *Psychosomatics, 38*(6), 548–557.

Poulton, A. A. (2005). Growth on stimulant medication; clarifying the confusion: A review. *Archives of Disease in Childhood, 90*, 801–806.

Poulton, A., Briody, J., McCorquodale, T., Melzer, E., Herrmann, M., Bauer, L. A., et al. (2012). Weight loss on stimulant medication: How does it affect body composition and bone metabolism? A prospective longitudinal study. *International Journal of Pediatric Endocrinology, 30*.

Rabiner, D. L., Anastopoulos, A. D., Costello, E. J., Hoyle, R. H., McCabe, S. E., & Swartzwelder, H. S. (2009). The misuse and diversion of prescribed ADHD medications by college students. *Journal of Attention Disorders, 13*(2), 144–153. doi:10.1177/1087054708320414.

Rawana, J. S., Morgan, A. S., Nguyen, H., & Craig, S. G. (2010). The relation between eating- and weight-related disturbances and depression in adolescence: A review. *Clinical Child and Family Psychology Review, 13*(3), 213–230.

Ruggiero, S., Rafaniello, C., Bravaccio, C., Grimaldi, G., Granato, R., Pascotto, A., et al. (2012). Safety of attention-deficit/hyperactivity disorder medications in children: An intensive pharmacosurveillance monitoring study. *Journal of Child and Adolescent Psychopharmacology, 22*, 415–422.

Schepis, T., & Hakes, J. K. (2011). Non-medical prescription use increases the risk for the onset and recurrence of psychopathology: Results from the national epidemiological survey on alcohol and related conditions. *Addiction, 106*, 2146–2155.

Schepis, T., & Krishnan-Sarin, S. (2008). Characterizing adolescent prescription misusers: A population based study. *Journal of the American Academy of Child and Adolescent Psychiatry, 47*(7), 745–754.

Striegel-Moore, R. H., Dohm, F. A., Kraemer, H. C., Taylor, C. B., Daniels, S., Crawford, P. B., et al. (2003). Eating disorders in white and black women. *The American Journal of Psychiatry, 160*, 1326–1331.

Substance Abuse and Mental Health Services Administration, Center for Behavioral Health Statistics and Quality. (July 2, 2012). *The DAWN report: Highlights of the 2010 drug abuse warning network (DAWN) findings on drug-related emergency department visits*. Rockville, MD: Substance Abuse and Mental Health Services Administration.

Substance Abuse and Mental Health Services Administration, Center for Behavioral Health Statistics and Quality. (January 24, 2013). *The DAWN report: Emergency department visits involving attention deficit/hyperactivity disorder stimulant medications*. Rockville, MD: Substance Abuse and Mental Health Services Administration.

Substance Abuse and Mental Health Services Administration. (2014). *Results from the 2013 National Survey on Drug Use and Health: Summary of National Findings, NSDUH Series H-48, HHS Publication No. (SMA) 14-4863*. Rockville, MD: Substance Abuse and Mental Health Services Administration.

Teter, C. J., McCabe, S. E., LaGrange, K., Cranford, J. A., & Boyd, C. J. (2006). Illicit use of specific prescription stimulants among college students. *Pharmacotherapy, 26*(10), 1501–1510.

Thompson, J. K., Heinberg, L. J., Altabe, M., & Tantleff-Dunn, S. (1999). *Exacting beauty: Theory, assessment, and treatment of body image disturbance*. Washington, DC: American Psychological Association.

Thompson, J. K., van den Berg, P., Roehrig, M., Guarda, A. S., & Heinberg, L. J. (2004). The sociocultural attitudes towards appearance scale-3 (SATAQ-3): Development and validation. *International Journal of Eating Disorders, 35*(3), 293–304. doi:10.1002/eat.10257.

Trenque, T., Herlem, E., Taam, M. A., & Drame, M. (2014). Methylphenidate off-label use and safety. *SpringerPlus, 3*, 286.

Vander Wal, J. S. (2012). The relationship between body mass index and unhealthy weight control behaviors among adolescents: The role of family and peer social support. *Economics & Human Biology, 10*(4), 395–404.

Wilens, T. E., Adler, L. A., Adams, J., Sgambati, S., Rotrosen, J., Sawtelle, R., et al. (2008). Misuse and diversion of stimulants prescribed for ADHD: A systematic review of the literature. *Journal of the American Academy of Child & Adolescent Psychiatry, 47*(1), 21–31.

Wu, L. T., Pilowsky, D. J., Schlenger, W. E., & Galvin, D. M. (2007). Misuse of methamphetamine and prescription stimulants among youths and young adults in the community. *Drug and Alcohol Dependence, 89*(2–3), 195–205. doi:10.1016/j.drugalcdep.2006.12.020.

Young, A. M., Glover, N., & Havens, J. R. (2012). Nonmedical use of prescription medications among adolescents in the United States: A systematic review. *Journal of Adolescent Health, 51*(1), 6–17.

Zachor, D. A., Roberts, A. W., Hodgens, J. B., Isaacs, J. S., & Merrick, J. (2006). Effects of long-term psychostimulant medication on growth of children with ADHD. *Research in Developmental Disabilities, 27*(2), 162–174. doi:10.1016/j.ridd.2004.12.004.

Zullig, K. J., & Divin, A. L. (2012). The association between non-medical prescription drug use, depressive symptoms, and suicidality among college students. *Addictive Behaviors, 37*(8), 890–899. doi:10.1016/j.addbeh.2012.02.008.

10

Commonly Prescribed Oral Anti-Obesity Medication and Alternative Anorectics

Julien S. Baker, Bruce Davies, and Michael R. Graham

Introduction

The mechanisms associated with being overweight have been used and are hoping to be used by the pharmaceutical industry to identify specific targets in an attempt to design pharmaceutical agents that can control body weight. Anti-obesity medicines act by decreasing energy intake, increasing energy expenditure or controlling lipid metabolism and fat stores. Despite the escalation in obesity over the last half century and our pre-occupation with our images, in the UK and the USA there are remarkably few medicines available which are effective in managing the

---

J.S. Baker (✉)
School of Science and Sport, University of the West of Scotland, ML3 0JB, Hamilton, Lanarkshire, UK

B. Davies
School of Science, University of South Wales, CF37 1DL, UK

M.R. Graham
Llantarnam Research Academy, NP44 3AF, UK

© The Editor(s) (if applicable) and The Author(s) 2016
M. Hall et al. (eds.), *Chemically Modified Bodies*,
DOI 10.1057/978-1-137-53535-1_10

problem. Since the 1950s, various medications were developed but either never made it to the market or were initially approved only to be withdrawn later, because of adverse health issues.

In the UK, the National Health Service (NHS) health professionals have very little training and education in University or Medical School on diet management other than recommended daily allowances of vitamins and minerals and the requirements of basic food groups. The treatment of NHS patients currently extends to the prescription of oral anti-obesity pharmacological medication, the offer of calorie controlled diet sheets, referral to local weight loss groups, and in certain areas referral, if appropriate, to a qualified trainer for exercise prescription. The National Institute for Health and Care Excellence (NICE) stipulate that prescription medicines can only be prescribed if the risks associated with obesity outweigh the risks of treatment (nice.org.uk).

The obesity epidemic that we are experiencing is a global phenomenon. In 2005 more than 1.6 billion adults over the age of 15 years were overweight and 400 million were obese (World Health Organisation 2014). By 2015 it has been predicted that more than 2.3 billion adults over the age of 15 years will be overweight and at least 700 million will be obese (World Health Organisation 2014).

The aetiology of obesity is complex. Genetic, environmental, and psychological factors are implicated in its causation. Obesity is a disorder of energy balance. When energy derived from food, chronically exceeds energy expenditure, the excess calories are stored as triglycerides in adipose tissue. Despite the marked fluctuations in daily food intake, body weight remains remarkably stable in most humans. In response to alterations in body adiposity, the brain triggers compensatory physiological adaptations that resist weight change. The causation of obesity has been suggested as being an unhealthy diet, excessive calorie intake over expenditure and a sedentary lifestyle. The reason for the global increase in obesity is complex and can only be explained by a combination of multiple factors. Numerous scientific studies within the last century have been conducted in an attempt to identify the reasons for the increase. A low resting metabolic rate has been suggested as one factor. However, obesity in the Pima Indian children compared with Caucasian children was shown not to be as a consequence of resting metabolic rate and that other factors such as diet and physical activity might be involved.

Prentice and Jebb (1995) suggested that modern inactive lifestyles were at least as important as diet in the aetiology of obesity and were in fact the dominant factor. According to the *"Physical Activity and Health"* report by the Surgeon General (1996), low levels of activity, resulting in fewer calories used than consumed, were contributing to the high prevalence of obesity in the USA (Eckel and Krauss 1998). A diet low in fat and unrefined carbohydrates was shown to be less fattening than a diet high in fat, indicating the importance of diet and quality of caloric intake, irrespective of physical activity (Astrup et al. 2000).

Dietary strategies which aim to reduce postprandial insulin response and increase fat oxidation, via a low-glycaemic index (GI) diet have been shown to have a prime position in the prevention and treatment of obesity and associated metabolic disorders (Munsters and Saris 2014). There is a suggestion that genetic predisposition may play a part in obesity and that the APOAF gene variation can modulate the effects of dietary fat on body mass index (BMI) and obesity risk (Corella et al. 2007).

Using exome sequencing Jiao et al. (2014) identified a low-frequency coding variant in the SYPL2 gene that was associated with morbid obesity. This gene may be involved in the development of excess body fat. However, no genetic explanation can explain how humans have become so fat so quickly. In the NHS, BMI is still currently the first method to determine if an individual is overweight. It is a weight to height ratio, measured in kilograms per metre^2 (kg/m^2). It is only a predictor of being overweight and body fatness and gives no indication of body fat distribution. It is ingrained in the system, because of the speed with which assessment can be made using a weighing scales and stadiometer. The classification of BMI with respect to the risks associated with being overweight and its management thereof, indicate that it will be used as the benchmark for the foreseeable future (WHO. Obesity: preventing and managing the global epidemic. Report of a WHO Consultation. WHO Technical Report Series 894. Geneva: World Health Organization 2000). See Table 10.1.

Table 10.1 The international classification of adult underweight, overweight, and obesity values according to BMI

Classification	BMI (kg/m^2)
	Principal values
Underweight	**<18.50**
Severe thinness	<16.00
Moderate thinness	16.00–16.99
Mild thinness	17.00–18.49
Normal range	**18.50–24.99**
Overweight	**≥25.00**
Pre-obese	25.00–29.99
Obese	**≥30.00**
Obese class I	30.00–34.99
Obese class II	35.00–39.99
Obese class III	≥40.00

BMI Classification

Body Mass Index (BMI) is a simple index of weight:height ratio that is commonly used to classify being underweight, overweight, and obesity levels in adults. It is defined as the weight in kilograms divided by the square of the height in metres (kg/m^2). For example, an adult who weighs 70 kg and whose height is 1.75 m will have a BMI of 22.9. BMI = 70 kg/(1.75 m^2) = 70/3.06 = 22.9 kg/m^2.

BMI values are age-independent and the same for both sexes. However, BMI may not correspond to the same degree of fatness in different populations due, in part, to different body proportions. The health risks associated with increasing BMI are continuous and the interpretation of BMI gradings in relation to risk may differ for different populations (Table 10.2).

In the USA, weight loss drugs approved by the Food and Drug Administration (FDA) and in the UK, weight loss drugs approved by NICE may only be used as part of a comprehensive weight loss program. This should include dietary therapy and physical activity, for patients with a BMI of ≥30 kg/m^2, with no concomitant obesity-related risk factors or diseases, and for patients with a BMI of ≥28 kg/m^2, with concomitant obesity-related risk factors or diseases (www.nhs.uk, 2014). The risk factors and diseases considered important enough to warrant pharmacotherapy at a BMI of 28–29.9 kg/m^2, are hypertension, dys-

Table 10.2 Drugs commonly used to treat obesity in the UK and USA

Drug and date of introduction	Mechanism of action	Weight reduction (kg/%)	Year of discontinuation from prescription or regulation	Side effects or cause of discontinuation
Orlistat (1990s)	Reducing fat absorption: lipase inhibitor	2.7 kg (2.9 %) at 1 year vs. controls (Padwal et al. 2004)	Still in use	Diarrhoea (steatorrheoa), flatulence, bloating
Ephedrine alkaloids (1900s) / Ephedra (Pre-Chinese Han dynasty)	Reducing food intake: sympathomimetic amine	Limited records	Regulated: 1997 (USA)/Withdrawn in 2004 (USA)	Cardiovascular and central nervous system symptoms resulting in high mortality
Tetra-iodothyronine and Tri-iodothyronine (Thyroid hormones) (1890s)	Increased basal metabolic rate	Limited records	1980	Hyperthyroidism, psychiatric symptoms, cardiac arrhythmias, sudden death
Clenbuterol (Awareness of drug use in sport since 1990s)	Reducing food intake: sympathomimetic amine	Limited records	Never licensed in UK or USA	Increase in risk of adverse cardiovascular and central nervous system symptoms
Sibutramine (1997)	Reducing food intake: combined norepinephrine and serotonin reuptake inhibitor	4.3 kg (15 %) at 1 year vs. controls (Padwal et al. 2004)	Withdrawn in 2010	Increase in risk of major adverse non-fatal cardiovascular and cerebrovascular events (and cardiovascular death)

(*continued*)

Table 10.2 (continued)

Drug and date of introduction	Mechanism of action	Weight reduction (kg/%)	Year of discontinuation from prescription or regulation	Side effects or cause of discontinuation
Phenylpropanolamine (1970)	Reducing food intake: sympathomimetic amine	Limited records	Withdrawn in 2000	Haemorrhagic stroke
Fenfluramine + Phentermine (1992)	Reducing food intake: sympathomimetic amine	Limited records	Withdrawn in 1997	Valvular heart disease
Lorcaserin 2012 (USA)	Reducing food intake: serotonin reuptake inhibitor	5 % at 2 years vs. controls (Hoy 2013)	Still in use	Headache, hypoglycaemia
Phentermine + Topiramate 2012 (USA)	Reducing food intake: sympathomimetic amine	10.2 kg at 1 year vs. controls (Gadde et al. 2011)	Still in use	Dizziness, paraesthesia, dry mouth, constipation
Rimonabant (2006)	Reducing food intake: selective CB1 receptor blocker	6.3 kg at 1 year vs. controls (Pi-Sunyer et al. 2006)	Withdrawn in 2009	Psychiatric disorders, depression and suicidal ideation

Abbreviations: United Kingdom = UK; United States of America = USA lipidaemia, coronary heart disease (CHD), type 2 diabetes, and sleep apnoea (National Institutes of Health, National Heart, Lung, and Blood Institute 1998) (Fig. 10.1).

Orlistat (tetrahydrolipstatin) is a drug designed to treat obesity. It is marketed as a prescription drug under the trade name Xenical by Roche in the UK, and is sold over-the-counter as Alli by GlaxoSmithKline (www.pharmacy2u.co.uk, 2014). It is currently the main prescription medicine used in the NHS used to treat obesity. It prevents the absorption of fats from the diet by acting as a lipase inhibitor. This reduces caloric intake. It is intended for use in conjunction with a supervised reduced-calorie controlled diet.

Orlistat is the saturated derivative of lipstatin, a potent natural inhibitor of pancreatic lipases isolated from the bacterium Streptomyces toxytricini (Borgström 1988). However, due to its stability, orlistat was chosen over lipstatin for development as an anti-obesity drug. The efficacy of orlistat in causing weight loss is limited. Data from short-term clinical trials over one year demonstrated that subjects who took orlistat lost 2.7 kg, or 2.9 % more body weight than those not taking the drug

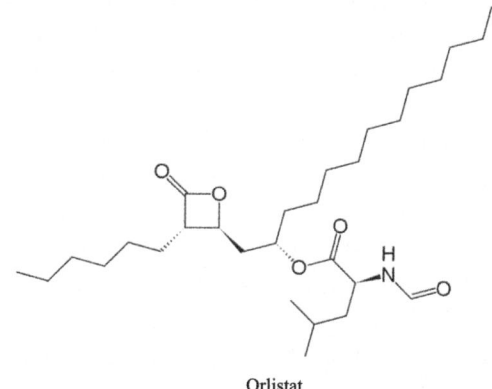

Orlistat

Chemical Formula: C29H53O5

Half life: 1–2 hours

Excretion: Faecal

Fig. 10.1 Orlistat (Xenical)

over the same period (Padwal et al. 2004). However, orlistat was shown to cause gastrointestinal (GI) side effects. Orlistat was found to reduce the incidence of type 2 diabetes, in obese people, with a BMI > 30 kg/m². After 4 years' treatment, the cumulative incidence of diabetes was 9.0 % with placebo and 6.2 % with orlistat, corresponding to a risk reduction of 37.3 % (Torgerson et al. 2004).

Mechanism of Action

Orlistat works by preventing around a third of the fat that is eaten from being digested. This undigested fat is not absorbed and is passed out with the faeces. With the correct diet this may avoid gaining weight, but does not necessarily cause weight loss. Therefore, a low fat diet and exercise is still recommended. Orlistat acts by binding covalently to the serine residue of the active site of gastric and pancreatic lipases, the enzymes that play an essential role in the digestion of dietary fat (triglycerides) in the GI tract, with very little activity against amylase, trypsin, chymotrypsin, and phospholipases. When administered with fat-containing foods, lipase activity is blocked by orlistat which partially inhibits hydrolysis of triglycerides, thus reducing the subsequent absorption of absorbable-free monoacylglycerides and free fatty acids which are excreted undigested. Only trace amounts of orlistat are systemically absorbed. The primary effect is local lipase inhibition within the GI tract after an oral dose. The primary route of elimination is through the faeces. Orlistat's pharmacological activity is dose-dependent. At the standard therapeutic dose (120 mg three times daily [t.d.s.] with main meals) administered in conjunction with a hypocaloric diet, the inhibition of fat absorption (approximately 30 % of ingested fat) contributes to an additional caloric deficit. The standard over-the-counter dose of 60 mg inhibits approximately 25 % of ingested fat. Higher doses do not produce more potent effects and lead to side effects (Guerciolini 1997).

Orlistat does not produce significant disturbances to GI physiological processes to or to the systemic balance of minerals and electrolytes, when a low fat diet is adhered. Also, orlistat does not affect the absorption and pharmacokinetics of drugs with a narrow therapeutic index or medicines frequently used by obese patients (Guerciolini 1997). Common side effects are fatty stools if a high fat diet is maintained (steatorrhoea), or more frequent urgent bowel motions, flatulence, and GI upset (Fig. 10.2).

Ephedrine is currently a prescription only medicine (POM) drug, despite being one of the most abused drugs in the health and fitness industry. It is a sympathomimetic amine which is still licensed for use in the NHS as a decongestant in much smaller doses, compared with the doses that are still being taken for the suppression of appetite. In previous years ephedrine was used as an appetite suppressant, to treat hypotension associated with anaesthesia and to treat myasthenia gravis (a neuromuscular disease that leads to fluctuating muscle weakness and fatigue). It was also used as a treatment for asthma as a bronchodilator, before the

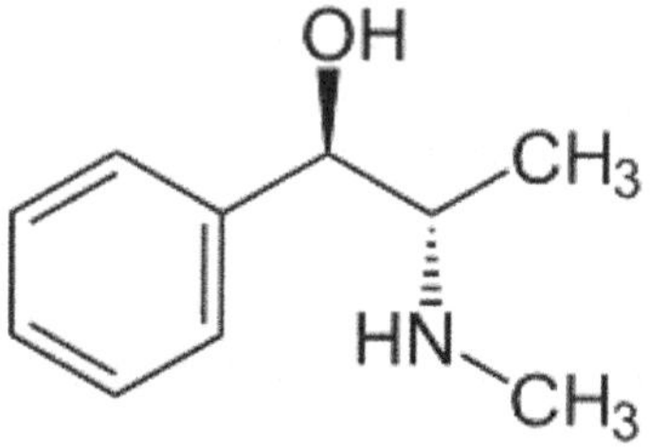

Ephedrine

Chemical Formula: $C_{10}H_{15}NO$

Pharmacokinetic data

Bioavailability: 85%

Metabolism: Hepatic

Half-life: 3–6 hours

Excretion: 22–99% (Renal)

Typical dosage per tablet: 15 mg, 25 mg, 30 mg

Fig. 10.2 Ephedrine

development of the selective beta agonists such as salbutamol. It has also been used to treat certain sleep disorders (narcolepsy), menstrual problems (dysmenorrhoea), and urinary problems (incontinence or enuresis).

In one study of 140 adverse events between 1997 and 1999, its use as a dietary supplement resulted in 47 % of individuals having cardiovascular symptoms and 18 % having central nervous system (CNS) symptoms. A high mortality of ten deaths necessitated that it should be treated with the utmost caution, allowing no more than 8 mg of ephedrine alkaloids per administrative dosage or 24 mg in a 24 hour period (Haller and Benowitz 2000). It has also been associated with other deaths (Theoharides 1997; Josefson 1996). Consequently ephedrine is rarely prescribed today because there are more specific treatments with far fewer side effects. Ephedrine should not be used in combination with other stimulant products (e.g. caffeine), other cough-and-cold products, or as a dietary supplement for the purpose of weight loss. Its use may increase the risk of potentially fatal side effects including: stroke, heart attack, seizures, or severe mental disorders.

Ephedrine is similar in molecular structure to the important neurotransmitter adrenaline. Chemically, it is an alkaloid with a phenethylamine skeleton found in various plants in the genus Ephedra (family Ephedraceae). It works mainly by increasing the activity of noradrenaline on adrenergic postsynaptic α- and β-receptors. It is most usually marketed as the hydrochloride or the sulphate salt. Ephedrine is able to cross the blood–brain barrier, and is a CNS stimulant similar to amphetamines, but less pronounced, as it releases noradrenaline and dopamine in the substantia nigra (Munhall and Johnson 2006).

The herb *Ephedra sinica* (Ma Huang), used in traditional Chinese medicine, contains ephedrine and pseudoephedrine (its diastereoisomer) as its principal active constituents. The same may be true of other herbal products containing extracts from other ephedra species. Pseudoephedrine is a commonly used and prescribed decongestant used in primary care to treat cough-and-cold complaints, but this has minimal CNS stimulant action and minimal appetite suppression compared with ephedrine.

Compared with prescription medicines, both in the NHS and the USA, there are dangers within the lesser controlled nutritional supplement business. Many manufacturers have used the manufacture of ephedrine as what was perceived as a legitimate business, to counterfeit more illicit drugs. In the USA, in January 1993 the state of California placed ephedrine and pseudoephedrine on its list of regulated chemicals, thus requiring that all transactions involving the sale or transfer of any amount of these chemicals be reported to the Department of Justice. Ephedra was not subjected to these rules because it was not specifically included on California's list of regulated chemicals. Therefore, in order to avoid exposing their illicit drug operations, clandestine laboratory operators manufactured ephedra (Andrews 1995). As of 2004 the US FDA had received over 18,000 reports of adverse effects of people using ephedrine and restrictions were imposed (Palamar 2011). Raw materials for the manufacture of ephedrine and traditional Chinese medicines are produced in China on a large scale. As of 2007, companies produced for export 13 million US$ worth of ephedrine from 30,000 tons of ephedra annually, which was ten times the amount used in traditional Chinese medicine. India is also a major exporter of ephedra products.

Recreational Use of Ephedrine

It is not uncommon for recreational sportspersons and individuals on diets to use stimulants when exercising. Ephedrine has been associated with dependence and as many as 25 % of 511 gymnasium attenders in the USA were users of the products. Extrapolating this to the general US population it was estimated that 2.8 million had used ephedrine in the previous 12 months (Kanayama et al. 2001). In the UK 44 % of 96 gymnasium attenders admitted to using ephedrine in the previous 12 months (Graham et al. 2006). There have been no new surveys since this period to identify whether the trend has changed.

A meta-analysis of short-term clinical trials of ephedrine and ephedra products demonstrated a short-term weight loss of approximately 0.9 kg/month, more than placebo. However, there was increased risk of psychiatric, autonomic, or GI symptoms, and heart palpitations and recommendations for its use could not be provided for long-term use (Shekelle et al. 2003). Ephedrine has been shown to stimulate thermogenesis in the brown adipose tissue (BAT), of lean but not obese humans (Carey et al. 2013). This suggests a concept that obese humans have only small amounts of BAT, which is inactive and that thermogenesis is assumed to take place mostly in the skeletal muscle.

Ephedrine is prohibited in sport, but is still legal to purchase for personal use both from chemists and from the Internet. Internet search engines allow a myriad of sites which will offer the products for sale (http://ephedrinewheretobuy.com, 2014). The problem with such products is that the quality control cannot be assured and contaminants may be present, which may compound adverse effects (Graham et al. 2009) (Figs. 10.3 and 10.4).

The thyroid hormones, triiodothyronine (T_3) and its prohormone, thyroxine (tetraiodothyronine, T_4), are tyrosine-based hormones produced by the thyroid gland that are responsible for the regulation of the basal metabolic rate, protein synthesis, regulation of longitudinal growth, neural maturation, and increases the cells' sensitivity to the catecholamines

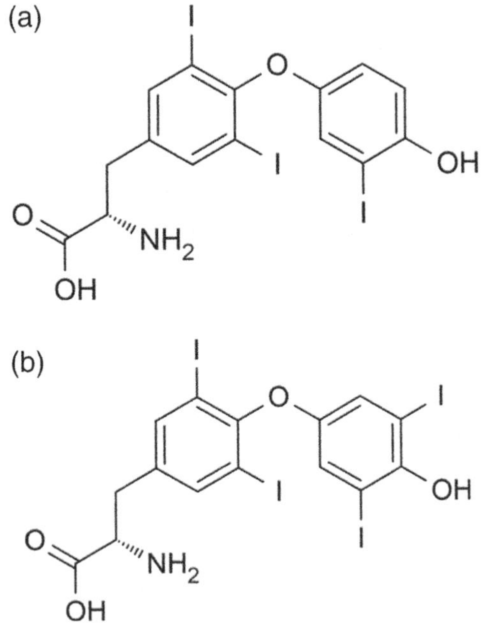

Fig. 10.3 (a) Triiodothyronine (T_3) (b) Tetraiodothyronine (T_4)

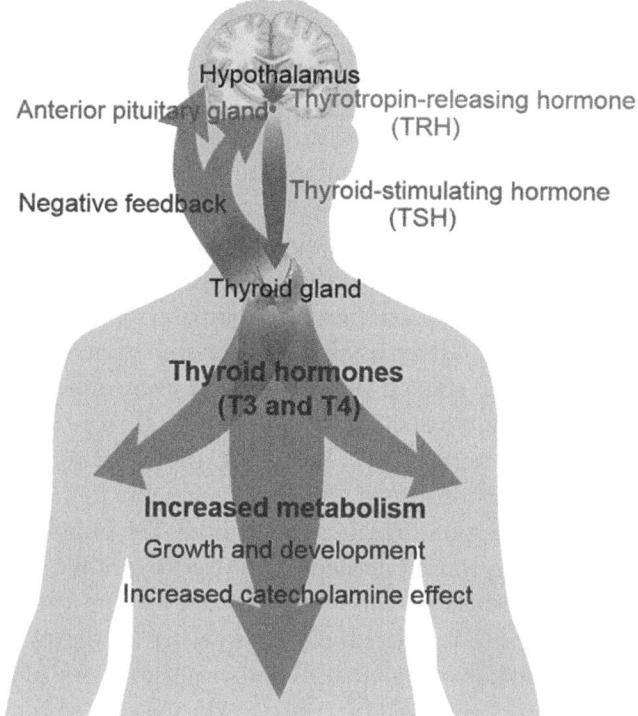

Fig. 10.4 Thyroid system

(adrenaline and nor-adrenaline). Thyroid hormones are essential for the development and differentiation of all cells of the human body. They also regulate protein, fat, and carbohydrate metabolism. Tetraiodothyronine, (T_4) and triiodothyronine, (T_3) are produced by the follicular cells of the thyroid gland. They are produced by attaching four and three iodine atoms to the ring structures of the tyrosine molecule, respectively. T_4 is believed to be a prohormone and reservoir for the most active and main thyroid hormone T_3. T_4 is converted as required in the tissues by iodothyronine deiodinase to T_3, which is more active than T_4.

Primary hypothyroidism is the most common pathological hormone deficiency, increases in incidence with age and occurs more often in women than in men. Globally, dietary iodine deficiency remains one of the most important causes of hypothyroidism (Roberts and Ladenson 2004).

Hypothyroidism can present with non-specific symptoms, such as weight gain, dyslipidaemia, hyponatraemia, hyperprolactinaemia, hyperhomocysteinaemia or with neuropsychiatric disorder. Severe untreated hypothyroidism can lead to heart failure, psychosis, and coma (Franklyn 2013). The diagnosis is confirmed by an elevated serum thyroid stimulating hormone (TSH) and low free T_4. Thyroxine replacement therapy, in deficiency, is highly effective and safe. Dysfunction of the thyroid axis is common in the general population and even more prevalent in the elderly, with an increased incidence of overt thyroid underactivity or over-activity (Boelaert 2013). Following the somatopause (andropause in males and menopause in females) there is a reduction in thyroid hormones and a corresponding increase in body fat. Subclinical (mild) thyroid dysfunction is more prevalent than overt hypothyroidism and is a condition characterized by abnormal (elevated) serum thyroid stimulating hormone (TSH) associated with normal serum thyroid hormone concentrations. The knowledge that hypothyroidism is one of the causes of obesity has been generalized by clinicians in the past to replace these hormones as a method of managing weight loss. In the UK, Harley Street clinicians were the main suppliers of thyroxine (T_4) as a slimming aid for overweight women in the sixties and seventies. However, excess thyroxine, taken by dieters in the absence of thyroid disease has resulted in iatrogenic thyrotoxicosis causing symptoms such as atrial fibrillation, cardiac arrhythmia, osteoporosis and in the extreme, sudden death (Franklyn 2013).

In the UK, one study identified that 10 % of 96 gymnasium attenders admitted to using T_3 or T_4 in the previous 12 months (Graham et al. 2006). Apart from sporadic case reports there appears to be no new epidemiological surveys identifying the extent of use of thyroid hormones. The case reports are often at the more serious end of the spectrum, where an individual requires hospital admission. In one case, a 32-year-old female was abusing levothyroxine as a slimming agent on advice of her gym instructor and had to be admitted to hospital with flaccid muscle weakness, as a result of hypokalaemia, after three months of thyroxine abuse (Chandey 2012). This required treatment with potassium supplementation and advice to discontinue use of thyroxine. The management of clinical hypothyroidism in clinical medicine is only with T_4 and not the combination of T_4 and T_3, despite the research of (Bunevicius et al. 1999), who demonstrated improved mood and neuropsychological function in combination therapy versus single therapy. Such research has not caught on in the health and fitness community, which may only lead to more adverse effects (Fig. 10.5).

Clenbuterol is a sympathomimetic amine, similar to ephedrine and a selective beta 2-adrenoceptor agonist used in Europe as a treatment for asthma, in humans and animals, where it is licensed for use by prescription. It is not licensed for use in the UK, where it is a controlled drug. It acts as a smooth muscle bronchodilator. It is most commonly taken orally as clenbuterol hydrochloride. It is chemically similar to salbutamol which is the recognized treatment for asthma in the UK (Nials et al. 1993). It is prohibited in sport but has gained a degree of notoriety as a weight loss drug and thermogenic agent, despite there being minimal supporting evidence that it has such effects. Past athletes, such as the German Katrin Krabbe have tested positive for clenbuterol and

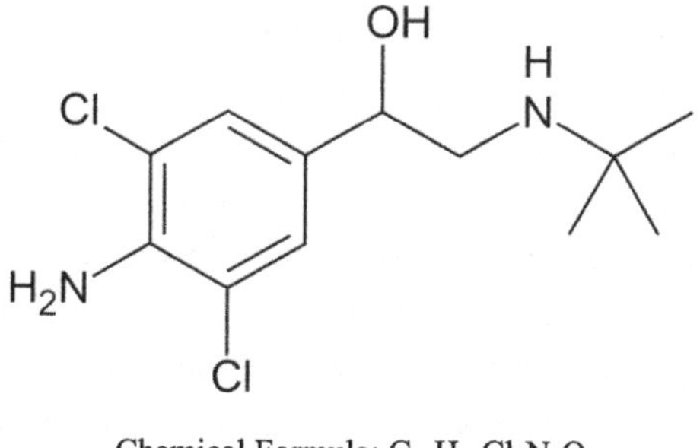

Chemical Formula: $C_{12}H_{18}Cl_2N_2O$
Half-life: 36–48 hours
Excretion: Faeces and urine

Fig. 10.5 Clenbuterol

been banned from competing (http://news.bbc.co.uk/sport1/hi/athletics/1960281, 2014). More recently in sport the four weight world champion Mexican boxer, Eric Morales was banned for two years for doping with clenbuterol (http://www.bbc.co.uk/sport/0/boxing/21908211, 2014). Its use by Hollywood celebrities for weight loss and the misinformation that is provided by the Internet has permitted it to gain an undeserved status allowing it to be purchased from unregulated sources (https://www.prbuzz.com/health-a-fitness, 2014). Excessive use over the recommended dose of about 120 µg three times per day can cause muscle tremors, headache, dizziness, and gastric irritation. Reported side effects include tachycardia, widened pulse pressure, tachypnoea, hypokalaemia, hyperglycaemia, arrhythmias (ST changes on electrocardiogram [ECG]), elevated cardiac troponin, elevated creatine phosphokinase (CPK), palpitations, chest pain, and tremor. In one study of misuse of clenbuterol by 11 of 13 subjects, the measured serum clenbuterol concentration was 2983 pg/mL post 4.5 mg ingestion, accounting for some or all the previous symptoms, which can persist for more than 24 hours post-cessation (Spiller et al. 2013). Internet sales of slimming agents have been adulterated with illicit compounds such as clenbuterol and other slimming agents and have been responsible for adverse events including fatalities (Parr et al. 2008; Rebiere et al. 2012).

Clenbuterol has contaminated the animal food chain as a growth-promoting and fat reducing drug, in countries where it was not licensed. It is not licensed for use in China, the USA, or the EU for food producing animals, but some countries have approved it for therapeutic use in food-producing animals. In 2011, China's largest meat producer, was exposed for using clenbuterol-contaminated pork in its meat products and its employees were prosecuted (http://news.xinhuanet.com, 2014). In Portugal, France, Spain, and China several outbreaks of food poisoning have been attributed to clenbuterol residue contamination of not pig organs and veal. Detection of the use of this product in animals is available in an attempt to prevent commercial organizations from contaminating the food industry (Pleadin et al. 2011). In the UK, 21 % of 96 gymnasium attenders admitted to using clenbuterol in the previous 12 months (Graham et al. 2006). This was increased from a previous study, conducted five years previously and nine years previously, respectively (Grace et al. 2001; Perry and Littlepage 1992) (Fig. 10.6).

In 1997 the prescription-only medicine, sibutramine was marketed as an adjunctive treatment for weight loss, with diet and exercise. Sibutramine is a centrally acting serotonin and noradrenaline reuptake inhibitor (SNRI) and works by appetite suppression (anorectic). It is similar in chemical structure to amphetamine. These two actions were identified as effective mechanisms of suppressing appetite. Fluoxetine and nisoxetine, selective reuptake inhibitors of serotonin and noradrenaline, respectively have no effect on food intake when given alone. They inhibit dietary intake when given in combination, however, demonstrating a synergistic interaction of those two monoamines in the control of eating and satiety, which is considered the two actions whereby sibutramine exerts its effect. Sibutramine also increases energy expenditure (thermogenesis) in rats, but it is not known if it has the same effect in humans (Heal et al. 1998). Sibutramine caused weight loss and improved lipid profile and glucose tolerance; however, an adverse effect was it also increased blood pressure (BP) and heart rate in clinical trials (James et al. 2000). Five sibutramine studies (three weight loss and two weight maintenance trials)

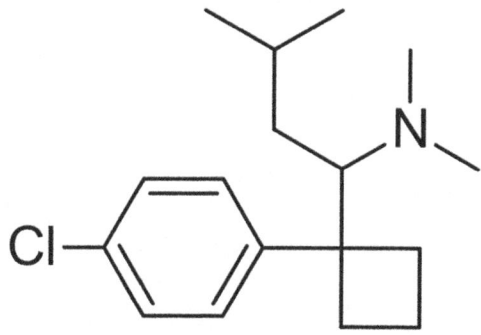

Chemical Formula: $C_{17}H_{26}ClN$

Half-life: 1 hour

Excretion: Faeces and urine

Fig. 10.6 Sibutramine

were compared with 11 orlistat studies. Patients on sibutramine experienced 4.3 kg weight loss (15 %) more than placebo, compared to 2.7 kg weight loss (12 %) of orlistat (14). At this time the modest increase in BP and heart rate were not considered a problem and certainly more favourable than orlistat which caused GI side effects. An ongoing randomized "Sibutramine Cardiovascular OUTcomes" (SCOUT) trial of 10,742 subjects, 84 % of whom had type 2 diabetes mellitus (DM) and additional co-morbidities demonstrated sibutramine and lifestyle modifications for 6 weeks resulted in small, but clinically relevant, median reductions in body weight, waist circumference, and BP. However, a small median increase in heart rate was recorded (Van Gaal et al. 2010). Subsequently, this study in 10,744 subjects with cardiovascular disease, DM, or both, found that sibutramine which was taken for 3.4 years, caused a greater rate of non-fatal cardiovascular and cerebrovascular events (James et al. 2010). The risk of a primary outcome event was 11.4 % in the sibutramine group versus 10 % in the placebo group (hazard ratio, 1.16; 95 % confidence interval [CI], 1.03 to 1.31; P = 0.02) and was considered significant enough to cause the voluntary withdrawal of sibutramine from the UK NHS market in January 2010 and the US market in October 2010. The mechanism of cardiovascular damage was believed to be an elevated rate pressure product (systolic blood pressure × heart rate mm.Hg × b.p.m.).

Sibutramine was developed and marketed by Knoll Pharmaceuticals and subsequently manufactured and marketed by Abbott Laboratories before its withdrawal from the market. It was sold under a variety of brand names including Reductil, Meridia, Siredia, and Sibutrex. In conjunction with the identification of its cardiovascular risks, sibutramine has been linked to multiple case histories of neuropsychiatric side effects (Nathan et al. 2011). Despite its withdrawal from the NHS market, it is still available through "legal" online websites (http://www.pharmacy2u.co.uk, 2014). The general population has been consuming anti-obesity medication for more than a century, resulting in an equally long history of unsafe drugs. Experimentation with dessicated thyroid gland began in the 1890s, but patients experienced side effects of hyperthyroidism.

The drug dinitrophenol (DNP) was first used for weight loss in 1933. Its side effects of blindness and hyperthermia caused fatalities and resulted in its withdrawal from the market in 1938 (Colman 2007). Combinations of amphetamine, thyroid hormone, and diuretics for weight loss and β-blockers and benzodiazepines to manage side effects were widely prescribed at private clinics from the 1940s to the 1970s, despite causing dozens of deaths before the authorities intervened and restricted their use (Cohen et al. 2012). However, in the USA and the UK, even after regulators limited their use by prescription they have continued to be supplied and taken as dietary supplements. One amphetamine, phenylpropanolamine, commonly found in appetite suppressants and cough-and-cold remedies has been considered an independent risk factor for haemorrhagic stroke in young women (Kernan et al. 2000).

Inadequately tested medications continued in the 1990s with fenfluramine and phentermine (Fen-Phen) which was the combination of two previously approved medications. Fenfluramine is a sympathomimetic amine that has an anorectic action mediated through the activation of serotonergic pathways in the brain. Fenfluramine promotes the rapid release of serotonin, inhibits its reuptake, with receptor-agonist activity, thus making serotonin more susceptible to metabolism and breakdown (Mitchell and Smythe 1990). Phentermine is an amphetamine derivative and a noradrenergic agent. Commonly used doses of these medications were 20 to 120 mg of fenfluramine per day and 15 to 30 mg of phentermine hydrochloride per day (Connolly et al. 1997). Despite the US FDA never approving the use of the combination, in 1996 more than 18 million prescriptions for "Fen-Phen" were issued in the USA (Connolly et al. 1997). In 1997, right-sided and left-sided valvular regurgitation and increased rates of pulmonary hypertension associated with "Fen-Phen" were identified (Connolly et al. 1997) and they were immediately withdrawn. Many patients filed lawsuits against drug manufacturers, resulting in billions of US$ claims. The history of obesity and its management by individual or combinations of pharmacotherapy agents has been fraught with negative adverse effects, rather than the positive effects of adipose tissue weight loss and the minimizing of the effects of obesity.

In 2012, the US FDA approved for weight loss, the selective serotonin agonist "lorcaserin", despite previous failed applications from 2009 onwards. Lorcaserin works as an anorectic in the same way that sibutramine works. It has been licensed for use only in the treatment of obesity for adults with a BMI ≥ 30 kg.m^{-2} or adults with a BMI of 27 kg.m^{-2} or greater who have at least one weight-related health condition, such as high blood pressure, type 2 diabetes mellitus, or high cholesterol. It has maintained weight loss of 5 % after two years' use compared with controls (Hoy 2013). This was the first approval since 1999. The drug is a controlled drug and can only be obtained by prescription in the USA, but is not available from the NHS in the UK. However it is available online and can be purchased with a credit or debit card (https://secure.theonlineclinic.co.uk, 2014). Also in 2012 the FDA approved the combination pill phentermine plus topiramate. Phentermine (PHEN) as previously stated is a noradrenergic agent and was withdrawn from the market, following cardiovascular side effects (Connolly et al. 1997). Topiramate (TPM) is a drug used as an anti-epileptic and antimigraine drug having effects on the CNS. It is thought to act as a γ-aminobutyric acid agonist that increases satiety.

In trials, the combination of the drug in low dose (3 mg PHEN plus 23 mg TPM) intermediate dose (PHEN 7·5 mg plus TPM 46 mg) and high dose (15 mg PHEN plus 92 mg TPM) have improved systolic blood pressure (SBP) and diastolic blood pressure (DBP), low density lipoprotein cholesterol (LDL-C) and high density lipoprotein cholesterol (HDL-C) levels, and fasting serum glucose relative to placebo. At a two year follow-up, phentermine plus topiramate reduced glycosylated haemoglobin (HbA$_1$C) in patients with DM (Garvey et al. 2012). HbA$_1$C serves as a marker for the average blood glucose levels, over the previous 8 weeks prior to the measurement, as this is the half-life of red blood cells. An average weight loss of 8.1 kg and 10.2 kg, respectively was attained at the end of 56 weeks with PHEN 7·5 mg plus TPM 46 mg, and PHEN 15 mg plus TPM 92 mg (Gadde et al. 2011). It is hoped that the lower dose of this combination, compared to the previously withdrawn medication dosages, will not lead to any long-term cardiovascular events. Continued scrutiny is required because of the effects of sympathomimetic stimulation, and current risk-factor analysis is insufficient to assess the safety in the long run.

Future Research

The neurotransmitters (serotonin, noradrenaline, dopamine, and histamine), peptides (neuromedin U, urocortin, bombesin, amylin, galanin), hormones (thyroid hormone, growth hormone), and cytokines (ciliary neurotrophic factor) play a very important part in feeding behaviour and energy expenditure (Morton et al. 2006). The brain controls energy homeostasis and body weight by integrating various metabolic signals. The research into the pharmacotherapy of obesity has been stimulated by the discovery of the effect leptin has on obesity. Leptin, which is an adipose-derived hormone, conveys critical information about peripheral energy storage and availability to the brain. Leptin decreases body weight by both suppressing appetite and promoting energy expenditure. Leptin resistance, a primary risk factor for obesity, may result from impairment in leptin transport, leptin signalling, and a sophisticated neuroendocrine system to control energy balance by constantly monitoring energy storage, availability from adipose tissue, and dietary consumption (Morris and Rui 2009). Leptin controls energy balance and body weight by regulating neuronal activity in the hypothalamus. Leptin decreases body weight both by suppressing appetite and by increasing energy expenditure. Leptin deficiency and genetic deficiency of functional leptin receptors (LEPR) results in morbid obesity and associated metabolic diseases. This has provided research into the exogenous administration of leptin, with little or no effect because of leptin resistance (Heymsfield et al. 1999; Foster-Schubert and Cummings 2006). In addition to controlling energy balance and body weight, leptin (in conjunction with the hormones ghrelin and insulin) also plays an important role in the regulation of mood and emotion and the rewards of food and of eating behaviour (Murray et al. 2014). Rimonabant was a drug introduced into the UK in 2006 as a long-term treatment for obesity. It had the unique mechanism of action of being a cannabinoid receptor blocker (Pi-Sunyer et al. 2006). It was known that cannabis use stimulated the appetite. Research trials showed weight loss and improvement in metabolic indices, but a long-term cardiovascular outcomes trial was terminated after revealing an increased rate of serious psychiatric side effects including suicide at mean follow-up of 14 months and the drug was withdrawn (Topol et al. 2010). This demonstrated the problems with bringing new drugs to the market to manipulate the metabolic system, in the management of obesity.

Conclusion

This short review demonstrates the risk to benefit ratio associated with attempting to control the metabolisms of the overweight and obese, with pharmacotherapy. There is considerable skepticism that the ingestion of one single drug or molecule can be responsible for controlling all the factors related to the cause of obesity. If one assesses the polypharmacy management of other hypokinetic diseases, society must understand that the management of weight is a multifactorial task that may benefit from pharmacotherapy, but that the best way to manage the problem is to prevent the problem occurring in the first instance. The main treatment for being overweight and changing anthropometry should still remain diet, nutritional management and physical exercise. This is a lifestyle change that the majority of individuals cannot implement.

References

Andrews, K. M. (1995). Ephedra's role as a precursor in the clandestine manufacture of methamphetamine. *Journal of Forensic Sciences, 40*, 551–560.

Astrup, A., Ryan, L., Grunwald, G. K., Storgaard, M., Saris, W., Melanson, E., et al. (2000). The role of dietary fat in body fatness: Evidence from a preliminary meta-analysis of ad libitum low-fat dietary intervention studies. *British Journal of Nutrition, 83*, 25–32.

Boelaert, K. (2013). Thyroid dysfunction in the elderly. *Nature Reviews Endocrinology, 9*, 194–204.

Borgström, B. (1988). Mode of action of tetrahydrolipstatin: A derivative of the naturally occurring lipase inhibitor lipstatin. *Biochimica et Biophysica Acta, 962*, 308–316.

Bunevicius, R., Kazanavicius, G., Zalinkevicius, R., & Prange Jr., A. J. (1999). Effects of thyroxine as compared with thyroxine plus triiodothyronine in patients with hypothyroidism. *The New England Journal of Medicine, 340,* 424–429.

Carey, A. L., Formosa, M. F., Van Every, B., Bertovic, D., Eikelis, N., Lambert, G. W., et al. (2013). Ephedrine activates brown adipose tissue in lean but not obese humans. *Diabetologia, 56,* 147–155.

Chandey, M. (2012). Thyroxine containing slimming agents, a threat to life. *Journal of Clinical and Diagnostic Research, 6,* 876–878.

Cohen, P. A., Goday, A., & Swann, J. P. (2012). The return of rainbow diet pills. *American Journal of Public Health, 102,* 1676–1686.

Colman, E. (2007). Dinitrophenol and obesity: An early twentieth-century regulatory dilemma. *Regulatory Toxicology and Pharmacology, 48,* 115–117.

Connolly, H. M., Crary, J. L., McGoon, M. D., Hensrud, D. D., Edwards, B. S., Edwards, W. D., et al. (1997). Valvular heart disease associated with fenfluramine-phentermine. *The New England Journal of Medicine, 337,* 581–588.

Corella, D., Lai, C. Q., Demissie, S., Cupples, L. A., Manning, A. K., Tucker, K. L., et al. (2007). APOA5 gene variation modulates the effects of dietary fat intake on body mass index and obesity risk in the Framingham Heart Study. *Journal of Molecular Medicine (Berlin), 85,* 119–128.

Eckel, R. H., & Krauss, R. M. (1998). American Heart Association call to action: Obesity as a major risk factor for coronary heart disease. AHA Nutrition Committee. *Circulation, 97,* 2099–2100.

Foster-Schubert, K. E., & Cummings, D. E. (2006). Emerging therapeutic strategies for obesity. *Endocrine Reviews, 27,* 779–793.

Franklyn, J. A. (2013). The thyroid—Too much and too little across the ages. The consequences of subclinical thyroid dysfunction. *Clinical Endocrinology, 78,* 1–8.

Gadde, K. M., Allison, D. B., Ryan, D. H., Peterson, C. A., Troupin, B., Schwiers, M. L., et al. (2011). Effects of low-dose, controlled-release, phentermine plus topiramate combination on weight and associated comorbidities in overweight and obese adults (CONQUER): A randomised, placebo-controlled, phase 3 trial. *Lancet, 377,* 1341–1352.

Garvey, W. T., Ryan, D. H., Look, M., Gadde, K. M., Allison, D. B., Peterson, C. A., et al. (2012). Two-year sustained weight loss and metabolic benefits with controlled-release phentermine/topiramate in obese and overweight adults (SEQUEL): A randomized, placebo-controlled, phase 3 extension study. *The American Journal of Clinical Nutrition, 95,* 297–308.

Grace, F. M., Baker, J. S., & Davies, B. (2001). Anabolic androgenic steroid (AAS) use in recreational gym users—A regional sample of the mid-glamorgan area. *Journal of Substance Use, 12*, 145–153.

Graham, M. R., Baker, J. S., & Davies, B. (2006). "Steroid" and prescription medicine abuse in the health and fitness community; A regional study. *European Journal of Internal Medicine, 17*, 479–484.

Graham, M. R., Ryan, P., Baker, J. S., Davies, B., Thomas, N. E., Cooper, S. M., et al. (2009). Counterfeiting in performance and image-enhancing drugs. *Drug Testing and Analysis, 1*, 135–142.

Guerciolini, R. (1997). Mode of action of orlistat. *International Journal of Obesity and Related Metabolic Disorders, 21*, S12–S23.

Haller, C. A., & Benowitz, N. L. (2000). Adverse cardiovascular and central nervous system events associated with dietary supplements containing ephedra alkaloids. *The New England Journal of Medicine, 343*, 1833–1838.

Heal, D. J., Aspley, S., Prow, M. R., Jackson, H. C., Martin, K. F., & Cheetham, S. C. (1998). Sibutramine: A novel anti-obesity drug. A review of the pharmacological evidence to differentiate it from D-amphetamine and D-fenfluramine. *International Journal of Obesity and Related Metabolic Disorders: Journal of the International Association for the Study of Obesity, 22*: S18–S28; discussion S29.

Heymsfield, S. B., Greenberg, A. S., Fujioka, K., Dixon, R. M., Kushner, R., Hunt, T., et al. (1999). Recombinant leptin for weight loss in obese and lean adults: A randomized, controlled, dose-escalation trial. *JAMA, 282*, 1568–1575.

Hoy, S. M. (2013). Lorcaserin: A review of its use in chronic weight management. *Drugs, 73*, 463–473.

James, W. P., Astrup, A., Finer, N., Hilsted, J., Kopelman, P., Rössner, S., et al. (2000). Effect of sibutramine on weight maintenance after weight loss: A randomised trial. STORM Study Group. Sibutramine Trial of Obesity Reduction and Maintenance. *Lancet, 356*, 2119–2125.

James, W. P., Caterson, I. D., Coutinho, W., Finer, N., Van Gaal, L. F., Maggioni, A. P., et al. (2010). Effect of sibutramine on cardiovascular outcomes in overweight and obese subjects. *The New England Journal of Medicine, 363*, 905–917.

Jiao, H., Arner, P., Gerdhem, P., Strawbridge, R. J., Näslund, E., Thorell, A., Hamsten, A. Kere, J. & Dahlman, I. (2014). Exome sequencing followed by genotyping suggests SYPL2 as a susceptibility gene for morbid obesity. *The European Journal of Human Genetics*, November 19 [Epub ahead of print].

Josefson, D. (1996). Herbal stimulant causes US deaths. *British Medical Journal, 312*, 1378–1379.
Kanayama, G., Gruber, A. J., Pope, H. G., Borowiecki, J. J., Jr., & Hudson, J. I. (2001). Over-the-counter drug use in gymnasiums: An under-recognized substance abuse problem? *Psychotherapy and Psychosomatics, 70*, 137–140.
Kernan, W. N., Viscoli, C. M., Brass, L. M., Broderick, J. P., Brott, T., Feldmann, E., et al. (2000). Phenylpropanolamine and the risk of hemorrhagic stroke. *The New England Journal of Medicine, 343*, 1826–1832.
Mitchell, P., & Smythe, G. (1990). Hormonal responses to fenfluramine in depressed and control subjects. *Journal of Affective Disorders, 19*, 43–51.
Morris, D. L., & Rui, L. (2009). Recent advances in understanding leptin signaling and leptin resistance. *American Journal of Physiology, Endocrinology and Metabolism, 297*, 1247–1259.
Morton, G. J., Cummings, D. E., Baskin, D. G., Barsh, G. S., & Schwartz, M. W. (2006). Central nervous system control of food intake and body weight. *Nature, 443*, 289–295.
Munhall, A. C., & Johnson, S. W. (2006). Dopamine-mediated actions of ephedrine in the rat substantia nigra. *Brain Research, 1069*, 96–103.
Munsters, M. J., & Saris, W. H. (2014). Body weight regulation and obesity: Dietary strategies to improve the metabolic profile. *Annual Review of Food Science and Technology, 5*, 39–51.
Murray, S., Tulloch, A., Gold, M. S., & Avena, N. M. (2014). Hormonal and neural mechanisms of food reward, eating behaviour and obesity. *Nature Reviews Endocrinology, 10*, 540–552.
Nathan, P. J., O'Neill, B. V., Napolitano, A., & Bullmore, E. T. (2011). Neuropsychiatric adverse effects of centrally acting antiobesity drugs. *CNS Neuroscience & Therapeutics, 17*, 490–505.
National Institutes of Health, National Heart, Lung, and Blood Institute. (1998). Clinical guidelines on the identification, evaluation, and treatment of overweight and obesity in adults: The evidence report. *Obesity Research, 6*, S51–S209.
Nials, A. T., Coleman, R. A., Johnson, M., Magnussen, H., Rabe, K. F., & Vardey, C. J. (1993). Effects of beta-adrenoceptor agonists in human bronchial smooth muscle. *British Journal of Pharmacology, 110*, 1112–1116.
Padwal, R., Li, S. K., & Lau, D. C. (2004). Long-term pharmacotherapy for obesity and overweight. *Cochrane Database Systematic Reviews*, (3):CD004094.
Palamar, J. (2011). How ephedrine escaped regulation in the United States: A historical review of misuse and associated policy. *Health Policy, 99*, 1–9.

Parr, M. K., Koehler, K., Geyer, H., Guddat, S., & Schänzer, W. (2008). Clenbuterol marketed as dietary supplement. *Biomedical Chromatography,* 22, 298–300.

Perry, H., & Littlepage, B. (1992). Dying to be big: A review of anabolic steroid use. *British Journal of Sports Medicine,* 4, 259–261.

Pi-Sunyer, F. X., Aronne, L. J., Heshmati, H. M., Devin, J., & Rosenstock, J. (2006). RIO-North America Study Group. Effect of rimonabant, a cannabinoid-1 receptor blocker, on weight and cardiometabolic risk factors in overweight or obese patients: RIO-North America: A randomized controlled trial. *JAMA: The Journal of the American Medical Association,* 295, 761–775.

Pleadin, J., Vulić, A., Mitak, M., Perši, N., & Milić, D. (2011). Determination of clenbuterol residues in retinal tissue of food-producing pigs. *Journal of Analytical Toxicology,* 35, 28–31.

Prentice, A. M., & Jebb, S. A. (1995). Obesity in Britain: Gluttony or sloth? *British Medical Journal,* 311, 437–439.

Rebiere, H., Guinot, P., Civade, C., Bonnet, P. A., & Nicolas, A. (2012). Detection of hazardous weight-loss substances in adulterated slimming formulations using ultra-high-pressure liquid chromatography with diode-array detection. *Food Additives & Contaminants. Part A, Chemistry, Analysis, Control, Exposure & Risk Assessment,* 29, 161–171.

Roberts, C. G., & Ladenson, P. W. (2004). Hypothyroidism. *Lancet,* 363, 793–803.

Shekelle, P. G., Hardy, M. L., Morton, S. C., Maglione, M., Mojica, W. A., Suttorp, M. J., et al. (2003). Efficacy and safety of ephedra and ephedrine for weight loss and athletic performance: A meta-analysis. *JAMA: The Journal of the American Medical Association,* 289, 1537–1545.

Spiller, H. A., James, K. J., Scholzen, S., & Borys, D. J. (2013). A descriptive study of adverse events from clenbuterol misuse and abuse for weight loss and bodybuilding. *Substance Abuse,* 34, 306–312.

Surgeon General (1996). Physical Activity and Health. http://www.cdc.gov/nccdphp/sgr/pdf/execsumm.pdf

Theoharides, T. C. (1997). Sudden death of a healthy college student related to ephedrine toxicity from a ma huang-containing drink. *Journal of Clinical Psychopharmacology,* 17, 437–439.

Topol, E. J., Bousser, M. G., Fox, K. A., Creager, M. A., Despres, J. P., Easton, J. D., et al. (2010). CRESCENDO investigators. Rimonabant for prevention of cardiovascular events (CRESCENDO): A randomised, multicentre, placebo-controlled trial. *Lancet,* 376, 517–523.

Torgerson, J. S., Hauptman, J., Boldrin, M. N., & Sjöström, L. (2004). Xenical in the prevention of diabetes in obese subjects (XENDOS) study: A randomized study of orlistat as an adjunct to lifestyle changes for the prevention of type 2 diabetes in obese patients. *Diabetes Care, 27,* 155–161.

Van Gaal, L. F., Caterson, I. D., Coutinho, W., Finer, N., Maggioni, A. P., Sharma, A. M., et al. (2010). SCOUT investigators. Weight and blood pressure response to weight management and sibutramine in diabetic and nondiabetic high-risk patients: An analysis from the 6-week lead-in period of the sibutramine cardiovascular outcomes (SCOUT) trial. *Diabetes, Obesity & Metabolism, 12,* 26–34.

World Health Organisation (2014). World Health Statistics. http://www.who.int/gho/publications/world_health_statistics/2014/en/

11

Peptide Hormones, Metformin and New-Wave Practices and Research Therapies

Michael R. Graham, Julien S. Baker, and Bruce Davies

Introduction

Human growth hormone (hGH) was isolated by Li and Papkoff (1956) and recombinant human growth hormone (rhGH) was synthesized by recombinant deoxyribonucleic acid (DNA) technology in the late 1970s (Goeddel et al. 1979). Subsequently, both amateur and professional athletes have been trying to extrapolate the benefits of replacement therapy in GH deficiency (GHD) to improve their cosmetic appearance and exercise performance (Salomon et al. 1989; Graham et al. 2009). Human GH first appeared in the underground doping literature in the early 1980s (Duchaine 1983). There are no certified statistics to show rhGH usage amongst athletes, nor the general population. The cases of rhGH abuse that have been identified in sport

---

M.R. Graham (✉) • B. Davies
School of Science & Sport, Llantarnam Research Academy, NP44 3AF, Cwmbran, UK

J.S. Baker
School of Science and Sport, University of the West of Scotland, ML3 0JB, Hamilton, Lanarkshire, UK

© The Editor(s) (if applicable) and The Author(s) 2016
M. Hall et al. (eds.), *Chemically Modified Bodies*,
DOI 10.1057/978-1-137-53535-1_11

are case histories of individuals who have been caught in possession at international tournaments. The possession of rhGH by the Chinese swimmers bound for the 1998 World Swimming Championships and similar problems at the Tour de France cycling event in 1998 suggested abuse at an elite level (Wallace et al. 1999). Latter day icons such as Arnold Schwarzenegger and sporting heroes such as Ben Johnson, Angella Issajenko, Dwain Chambers, Kelly White, Tim Montgomery, Marion Jones, and Lance Armstrong have all admitted doping with rhGH, to judicial enquiries, citing the speed up of their recovery times and enhancement of their physiques, not necessarily their performance in sport. Because of the difficulty in detecting rhGH use, up until this time any individual who was caught doping, tested positive for drugs other than rhGH. Two approaches have been investigated to detect rhGH abuse: the first is based on the detection of different pituitary GH isoforms and the ratio of 22-kDa isoform to total GH (Wu et al. 1999). The second test relies on measurement of GH-dependent markers, namely insulin-like growth factor-I (IGF-I) and N-terminal propeptide of type III procollagen (P-III-P) which would appear to increase in a dose-dependent manner in response to GH administration (Powrie et al. 2007; Erotokritou-Mulligan et al. 2010). Both methodologies have been approved by the World Anti-Doping Agency (WADA) and have led to the detection of a number of athletes misusing GH (Holt 2013).

The difficulty of identifying abuse in sport was highlighted in 2011. An Estonian Olympic gold medal winning skier, tested positive for rhGH. However, on challenging the finding in the Court of Arbitration for Sport (CAS) he was subsequently acquitted in 2013. The court was not convinced that the threshold limits for considering an adverse analytical finding were sufficiently reliable to uphold the doping conviction, despite confirming the validity of the test. A financial award was ordered by CAS to the skier (http://www.tas-cas.org/d2wfiles/document/6633/5048/0/256620).

For rhGH detection, both IGF-I and P-III-P are more stable than GH, which is why the World Anti-Doping Authority (WADA) use "serum profiling" of athletes, which is called a "biological passport" to detect the use of rhGH and rhIGF-I (Erotokritou-Mulligan et al. 2011). At the 2012 London Olympic and Paralympic games this "serum biological passport" analysis, resulted in the disqualification of two

Russian paralympic powerlifters, who admitted injecting GH after an adverse analytical finding (http://www.paralympic.org/press-release/latest-testing-methods-result-suspension-two-russian-powerlifters-anti-doping). Unequivocal detection, as is available for xenobiotic testosterone, however, is still problematic and ongoing (http://www.ukad.org.uk/news/article/uk-research-leads-to-new-growth-hormone-test). The prevalence of recombinant human (rh)IGF-I use is probably much lower than for rhGH because, it has only become freely available, via the Internet, through recombinant DNA technology in the last decade. RhIGF-I, has approval for use in humans to treat growth failure in children with severe primary IGF-I deficiency or with GH gene deletion who have developed neutralizing GH anti-bodies. One of the products is rhIGF-I, and the other product is recombinant human rhIGF-I bound to its major binding protein, IGFBP-3 (rhIGF-I LR3), which prolongs the half-life of IGF and counteracts adverse effects—for example, hypoglycaemia, associated with the administration of rhIGF-I (Kemp 2007).

The insulin-like growth factors (IGFs) are proteins with high-sequence similarity to insulin. They are part of a complex system that cells use to communicate with their environment. IGF-1 is mainly secreted by the liver and is induced by GH secretion (Le Roith et al. 2001). IGF-1 induces cell proliferation and is thought to inhibit cell death (apoptosis) (O'Reilly et al. 2006). It consists of 70 amino acids in a single chain with three intra-molecular disulphide bridges. IGF-1 has a molecular weight of 7649 Da. It displays homology to proinsulin, the precursor of insulin (Rinderknecht and Humbel 1978). IGF-1 mediates some of the metabolic actions of GH and has both GH-like and insulin-like actions. Both GH and IGF-1 have a net anabolic effect enhancing whole body protein synthesis, improving anthropometry in GHD. Both hormones have been used in catabolism and have been effective in counteracting the protein wasting effects of glucocorticoids. IGF-1 administration improves insulin sensitivity, whereas GH therapy can cause compensatory hyperinsulinaemia. IGF-2 is thought to be a primary growth factor required for early development while IGF-1 expression is required for achieving maximal growth. Factors that are known to cause variation in the levels of IGF-1 in the circulation, include genetic make-up, diurnal variation, age, sex, exercise status, stress levels, nutrition and disease state. IGF-1 has an involvement in regulating neurogenesis, myelination, synaptogenesis, and dendritic branching and neuroprotection after neuronal damage. The IGF-1 level reflects the secretory activity of GH and is a marker for identification of normal GH production (Mauras and Haymond 2005). Levels of IGF-1 are at their peak during late adolescence and decline throughout adulthood, mirror imaging GH (Milani et al. 2004). The concomitant administration of rhGH and rhIGF in GH resistant states has been shown to be synergistic and have effects that are far greater than either alone (Mauras and Haymond 2005). Athletes believe that the combination is more powerful than double of either alone and lower doses of both will limit detection. Such beliefs appear to be supported by contemporary research (Mauras and Haymond 2005; Holt 2013). There currently appears to be no technology to detect IGF-I abuse, but a similar approach as the GH-dependent marker test, is currently being evaluated by the GH-2000 and GH-2004 research teams.

The cases of insulin misuse that have been published are those that have been admitted to hospital following accidental overdose and the effects of excess exogenous insulin are well reported (Konrad et al. 1998; Evans and Lynch 2003). Dawson (2001) reported that 10 % of 450 patients attending his needle exchange programme self-prescribed insulin for non-therapeutic purposes. The covert nature of its abuse precludes exact figures. Prior to the availability of IGF-I, short acting insulin appeared to have been used in a random manner to increase muscle bulk in bodybuilders, weight lifters, and power lifters (Sonksen 2001). A questionnaire survey by Graham et al. (2006) demonstrated an increase in the abuse of insulin from 8 %, to 14 %, and an increase in the abuse of growth hormone from 6 %, to 24 %, in comparison to a survey conducted by Grace et al. (2001). The detection of insulin is similar to that of GH. Insulin is a naturally occurring pulsatile peptide hormone. There are no methods to detect endogenous insulin abuse but such availability in sport is non-existent. Urinary mass spectroscopy can detect the presence of analogue insulin. Liquid chromatography/mass spectrometry produces characteristic product spectra obtained from the analogues that differ from human insulin, permitting detection (Holt 2013; Thevis et al. 2006; Thomas et al. 2007).

United Kingdom Law and Ethical Consideration

Growth hormone (somatotropin) and insulin-like growth factor (IGF)-I are controlled drugs 'Class C' under the Misuse of Drugs Act, 1971, and both are defined as a 'Schedule 4 drug' under the Misuse of Drugs Regulations, 2001. The commission of offences in relation to the drug comes under the umbrella of the misuse of drugs act. Possession of this drug for self-administration is not a criminal offence, outside sport. However, testing positive and receiving financial reward for professional participation in sport is illegal.

Insulin and Metformin are prescription-only medicines. The commission of offences in relation to the drug comes under the Medicines Act, 1968. Possession of these medicines for self-administration is not a criminal offence. All of the medicines are banned by the World anti-doping authority (WADA) but appear to be an accepted part of amateur and professional bodybuilding. The International Olympic Committee (IOC) has very specific guidelines on the taking of insulin. It permits only the treatment of athletes with certified insulin-dependent diabetes and considers it an offence if any other competitor (i.e. a non-insulin dependent diabetic) is found to be in possession.

Physiology of Growth Hormone and IGF-I

A cascade of interacting transcription factors and genetic elements normally determines the ability of the somatotroph cells in the anterior pituitary to synthesize and secrete the polypeptide human growth hormone (hGH). The development and proliferation of somatotrophs are largely determined by a gene called the Prophet of Pit-1 (PROP1), which controls the embryonic development of cells of the Pit-1 (POU1F1) transcription factor lineage. Pit-1 binds to the growth hormone promoter within the cell nucleus, a step that leads to the development and proliferation of somatotrophs and growth hormone transcription. Once translated, growth hormone is secreted as a 191-amino-acid, 4-helix bundle protein (70–80 %) and a less abundant 176-amino-acid form (20–30 %), (Baumann 1991). This enters the circulation in pulsatile fashion under dual hypothalamic control through hypothalamic-releasing and hypothalamic-inhibiting hormones that traverse the hypophysial portal system and act directly on specific somatotroph surface receptors (Melmed 2006).

Growth hormone releasing hormone (GHRH) induces the synthesis and secretion of growth hormone, and somatostatin suppresses the secretion of growth hormone. Growth hormone is also regulated by ghrelin, a growth hormone secretagogue–receptor ligand, that is synthesized mainly in the gastrointestinal tract (Kojima et al. 1999). In healthy persons, the GH level is usually undetectable (<0.2 μg.L^{-1}) throughout most of the day. There are approximately ten intermittent pulses of growth hormone per 24 hours, most often at night, when the level can be as high as 30 μg.L^{-1} (Melmed 2006). Fasting increases the secretion of growth hormone, whereas ageing and obesity are associated with suppressed secretory bursts of the hormone (Iranmanesh et al. 1991). The action of growth hormone is mediated by a growth hormone receptor, which is expressed mainly in the liver and in cartilage and is composed of preformed dimers that undergo conformational change when occupied by a growth hormone ligand, promoting signalling (Brown et al. 2005).

Growth hormone activates the growth hormone receptor, to which the intracellular Janus kinase 2 (JAK2) tyrosine kinase binds. Both the receptor and JAK2 protein are phosphorylated, and signal transducers and activators of transcription (STAT) proteins bind to this complex. STAT proteins are then phosphorylated and translocated to the nucleus, which initiates transcription of growth hormone target proteins (Argetsinger et al. 1993). Intracellular growth hormone signalling is suppressed by several proteins, especially the suppressors of cytokine signalling (SOCS). In conjunction with GH, IGF-I has varying differential effects on protein, glucose, lipid, and calcium metabolism, and therefore, body composition (Mauras et al. 2000). Direct effects result from the interaction of GH with its specific receptors on target cells. In the adipocyte, GH stimulates the cell to break down triglyceride and suppresses its ability to uptake and accumulate circulating lipids. Indirect effects are mediated primarily by IGF-I. Many of the growth promoting effects of GH, are due to the action of IGF-I on its target cells. In most tissues, IGF-I has local autocrine and paracrine actions, but the liver actively secretes IGF-I and its binding proteins, into the circulation. Little is known about the expression of skeletal muscle-specific isoforms of IGF-I gene in response to exercise in humans, nor the influence of age and physical training status. Greig et al. (2006) reported that a single bout of isometric exercise stimulated the expression of mRNA for the IGF-I splice variants IGF-IEa and IGF-IEc (mechano growth factor (MGF) within 2.5 hours, which lasts for at least 2 days after exercise.

Liu et al. (2003) examined the effects of rhGH on myostatin (a growth inhibitory protein) regulation in GHD. Skeletal muscle biopsies from the vastus lateralis were performed at 6-monthly intervals during 18 months of treatment. Myostatin messenger ribonucleic acid (mRNA) expression was significantly inhibited to 31 % of control by rhGH. The inhibitory effect of GH on myostatin was sustained after 18 months of rhGH treatment. These effects were associated with significantly increased lean body mass (LBM) after 18 months.

IGF-I's primary action is mediated by binding to its specific receptor, the insulin-like growth factor 1 receptor (IGF1R), which is present on many cell types in many tissues. Binding to the IGF1R, a receptor tyrosine kinase, initiates intracellular signalling; IGF-1 is one of the most potent natural activators of the AKT signalling pathway, a stimulator of cell growth and proliferation, and a potent inhibitor of programmed cell death (O'Reilly et al. 2006). Specific binding proteins (IGFBPs) regulate the function of IGF-I. Approximately 95 % is bound in a ternary complex of IGF-I, IGFBP-3 and an acid-labile subunit (Holt and Sönksen 2008). The half-life of IGF-I bound in a ternary complex is 12 to 15 hours, much greater than free IGF-I, which is only several minutes and very similar to GH (Guler et al. 1989). The half-life can currently be prolonged when IGF-I is administered as a complex with IGFBP-3 between 15 to 19 hours after the injection of the complex, and a single injection can be effective in increasing IGF-I concentrations for a 24 hour period (Camacho-Hübner et al. 2006). The application to abuse in sport or the health and fitness industry is all too apparent. See Fig. 11.1.

The side effects associated with excess rhGH administration are well documented and may affect any individual misusing it (Melmed 2006).

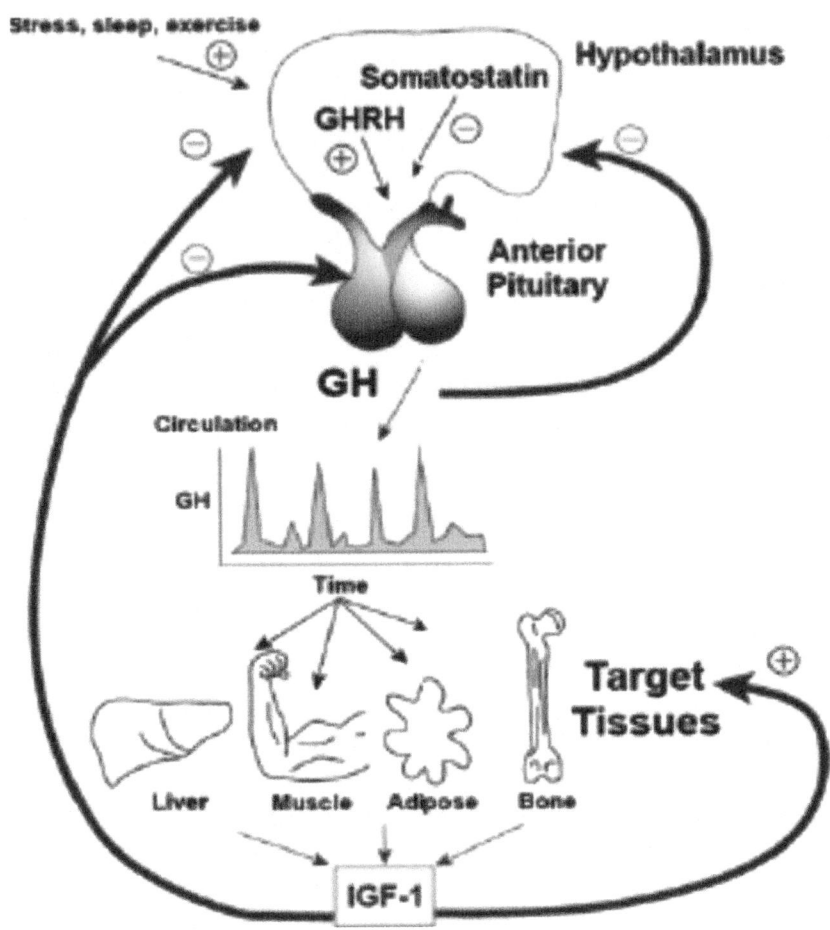

Fig. 11.1 The GH–IGF axis and regulation of GH and IGF-I synthesis and secretion

Anecdotal evidence suggests that many athletes take much higher doses than those used therapeutically, which may lead to features of acromegaly (gigantism) if use is prolonged. Effects can include headache, extracellular fluid retention, hypertension, diabetes mellitus, cardiovascular disease, and cardiomyopathy. The side effects of excess rhIGF-I administration, mirror those of rhGH excess, except it does not lead to diabetes, but may cause hypoglycaemia (Mauras and Haymond 2005).

Physiology of Insulin

Insulin is a 2 chain (30 & 21 amino-acids) polypeptide hormone (51 Amino-acids, Molecular weight 5808) synthesized and secreted by the Beta-cells of the islets of Langerhans in the pancreas gland. Insulin acts in a stimulatory and an inhibitory manner (Schafer 1916). It stimulates the translocation of glucose transporters 'Glut 4' from the cytoplasm of muscle and adipose tissue to the cell membrane. Insulin exhibits both inhibitory and excitatory actions via the same receptor. In experiments carried out on rat adipose tissue, in vitro insulin simultaneously inhibits lipolysis (the release of glycerol from stored triglyceride) and stimulates lipogenesis (formation of stored triglyceride from glucose). Thus its anabolic action is due to two mechanisms working synergistically (see Thomas et al. 1979).

Insulin stimulates the translocation of 'Glut 4' glucose transporters from the cytoplasm of muscle and adipose tissue to the cell membrane. This increases the rate of glucose uptake to values greater than in the basal state without insulin, shown in isolated adipocytes from rats. Insulin exhibits both inhibitory and excitatory actions via the same receptor.

Insulin increases glucose metabolism more through reducing free fatty acid (FFA) and ketone levels than it does through recruiting more glucose 'transporters' (GLUTs) into the muscle cell membrane. There are at least six types of these protein carriers (GLUTs) and they tend to be tissue-specific. In the case of muscle, the transporter is called 'Glut 4'. It is normally present in excess in the cell membrane even in the absence of insulin but is not rate limiting for glucose entry into the cell (Sonksen 2001). However, insulin does have a direct action recruiting more glucose transporters into muscle cell membranes. This facilitates glucose uptake which is reflected as an increase in the metabolic clearance rate (MCR) of glucose. The entry of a water-soluble substrate such as glucose across an impermeable lipid bi-layer into a cell requires the GLUT specific transport mechanism. Glucose transport into the cell is mainly determined by the concentration gradient between the extracellular fluid and the intracellular 'free' glucose. 'Free' glucose is very low inside the cell as it is immediately phosphorylated. In uncontrolled diabetes, particularly where there is a high concentration of FFA and ketones, glycolysis is inhibited, phosphorylation of 'free' glucose stops and intracellular 'free' glucose rises. Insulin recruits more transporters into the cell membrane from an intracellular pool. This increases the rate of glucose entry for a given glucose concentration and this is reflected in vivo by an increase in the MCR of glucose. Thus MCR is an in vivo measure of substrate transporter activity (Boroujerdi et al. 1995).

There are a sufficient number of glucose transporters in all cell membranes at all times to ensure enough glucose uptake to satisfy the cell's respiration, even in the absence of insulin. Insulin increases the number of these transporters in some cells but glucose uptake is never truly insulin dependent (Sonksen 2001). When insulin is given to patients with uncontrolled diabetes it switches off a number of metabolic processes (lipolysis, proteolysis, ketogenesis, and gluconeogenesis) by a similar inhibitory action. The result is that free FFA concentrations fall effectively to zero within minutes and ketogenesis inevitably stops through lack of substrate. It takes some time for the ketones to clear from the circulation, as they are water and fat soluble and distribute within body water and body fat. Both ketones and FFA compete with glucose as energy substrate at the point of entry into the Krebs cycle. Glucose metabolism increases as FFAs and ketone levels fall (Sonksen 2001).

The Effects of Growth Hormone on Anthropometry

RhGH administration has therapeutic value as a replacement therapy for GHD adults increasing lean mass and reducing total and visceral fat (Johannsson et al. 1997; Carroll et al. 1998). RhGH treatment increased LBM, decreased total cholesterol and LDL-cholesterol and increased HDL-cholesterol and results were sustained after 15 years, in A-OGHD (Elbornsson et al. 2013).

Effects in Healthy Individuals

GH secretion (and IGF-I) availability diminishes with age, 14 % per decade (Iranmanesh et al. 1991). The first researchers experimented on athletes using biosynthetic methionyl hGH (met-hGH), consisting of 192 amino-acids, as opposed to recombinant hGH (191 amino acids). Met-hGH (2.67 mg (~8 IU) 3 days per week) for 6 weeks in 8 well-trained exercising adults (22–33 years of age) trained with progressive resistance exercise who maintained a high-protein diet significantly decreased body fat and significantly increased LBM (Crist et al. 1988). Rudman et al. (1991) demonstrated that rhGH administration also benefitted elderly men, decreasing adiposity and increasing LBM (principally muscle). Muscle protein turnover and increases in muscle mass can occur over short periods of time (days) and can be measured indirectly using techniques such as hydrostatic weighing or dual X-Ray absorptiometry. RhGH administration (0.03 mg.kg^{-1} of body weight (7.2 IU x 3.week^{-1}), for 6 months in 52 healthy men (75 years, 80 kg) with well-preserved functional ability, but low baseline IGF-I levels, significantly increased LBM, on average by 4.3 % (Papadakis et al. 1996). RhGH significantly increased the myosin heavy chain (MHC) 2X isoforms (Lange et al. 2002). This has been regarded as a change into a more youthful MHC composition, possibly induced by the rejuvenation of systemic IGF-I levels.

Healy et al. (2003) has shown that rhGH exerts an anabolic effect both at rest and during exercise in endurance-trained athletes, measuring whole body leucine turnover. Healy et al. (2006) showed that plasma levels of glycerol and free fatty acids and glycerol rate of appearance (Ra) at rest and during and after exercise increased during rhGH treatment compared with placebo. Glucose Ra and glucose rate of disappearance (Rd) were greater after exercise during rhGH treatment compared with placebo. Resting energy expenditure and fat oxidation were greater under resting conditions during rhGH treatment compared with placebo. Thirty healthy individuals (15 men and 15 women), age range 18–35 received rhGH (0.033 mg.kg^{-1}.day^{-1} (0.1 IU.kg^{-1}.day^{-1}); n = 10) or rhGH (0.067 mg.kg^{-1}.day^{-1} (0.2 IU.kg^{-1}.day^{-1}); n = 10) or placebo (n = 10) for

1 month. Body fat decreased significantly by 6.6 %, IGF-I significantly increased by 134 %, body weight significantly increased by 2.7 %, fat free mass significantly increased by 5.3 %, total body water significantly increased by 6.5 % and extracellular water (ECW) significantly increased by 9.6 % (Ehrnborg et al. 2005).

The interaction of GH and 11ßhydroxysteroid dehydrogenase (11ßHSD1 and 11ßHSD2) has been suggested in the pathogenesis of central obesity, in 30 men (aged 48–66 years) with abdomino-visceral obesity. After 6 weeks rhGH, 11ßHSD1 significantly decreased. After 9 months rhGH, 11ßHSD2 significantly increased. Between 6 weeks to 9 months glucose disposal rate increased and visceral fat mass decreased. Changes in 11ßHSD1 activity correlated with body composition and insulin sensitivity. However, the authors considered that the data could not support the hypothesis that long-term (9 months) metabolic effects of GH are mediated through its action on 11ßHSD 1 and 2 (Sigurjonsdottir et al. 2006). The relevance of these effects for cosmetic enhancement in middle age cannot be excluded.

The Effects of Different Dosages of rhGH

Effects of rhGH have been studied at greater than physiological dosages, and have resulted in serum concentrations of IGF-I that are at least twice normal (Yarasheki et al. 1995). There have been significant physiological effects: increased lipolysis, altered carbohydrate metabolism, activation of the renin-angiotensin system, and water retention. Such effects will improve cosmetic appearance by redistributing subcutaneous fat from central to peripheral deposits (Graham et al. 2008).

The Effects of Growth Hormone on Thyroid Function

The thyroid gland controls how quickly the body uses energy, makes proteins, and controls how sensitive the body is to other hormones. It participates in these processes by producing thyroid hormones, the principal ones being triiodothyronine (T_3) and tetraiodothyronine (thyroxine or T_4). These hormones regulate the growth and rate of function of many other systems in the body. T_3 and T_4 are synthesized from iodine and tyrosine. The thyroid also produces calcitonin, which plays a role in calcium homeostasis. Hormonal output from the thyroid is regulated by thyroid-stimulating hormone (TSH) produced by the anterior pituitary, which itself is regulated by thyrotropin-releasing hormone (TRH) produced by the hypothalamus.

GH influences thyroid function and anatomy. The effects of GHD are difficult to assess, because hypopituitary subjects who lack GH often also have a partial or complete deficit of thyroid stimulating hormone (TSH). RhGH is known to increase the metabolism of T_4, enhancing the conversion of T_4 to T_3 where T_4 was significantly lowered by 8 %, T_3 was significantly increased by 21 %, and TSH was significantly decreased by 54 %, after 4 days of low dose rhGH administration (0.125 mg.day^{-1} (0.4 IU.day^{-1}) (Grunfeld et al. 1988). The work of Wyatt et al. (1998) demonstrated that T_4 was unaltered after 12 months of rhGH replacement therapy.

Wyatt et al. (1998) showed that shifts in thyroid hormone levels are very common during the first year of GH therapy in children who are initially euthyroid. Baseline TSH, T_4, free T_4, reverse(r)T_3 and T_3 levels were normal, with negative anti-thyroid antibodies. By one month, there were significant decreases in T_4, free T_4 index and rT_3, and significant increases in T_3 and the T_3/T_4 ratio. The changes from baseline values were greatest at one month, but showed a gradual return to baseline from three to twelve months. There were no clinical signs of hypothyroidism. T_4 supplementation is seldom needed in such patients. Portes et al. (2000) demonstrated that long-term rhGH replacement therapy in GHD significantly decreases serum free T_4 and rT_3 levels and increases serum T_3 levels. These changes are independent of TSH and result from increased peripheral conversion of T_4 to T_3. GHD does not induce hypothyroidism, but simply reveals previously unrecognized cases whose serum free T_4 values fall in the low range during rhGH replacement.

Porretti et al. (2002) showed that GHD masks a state of central hypothyroidism, in a consistent number of adult patients. Therefore, during rhGH treatment, monitoring of thyroid function is mandatory to start

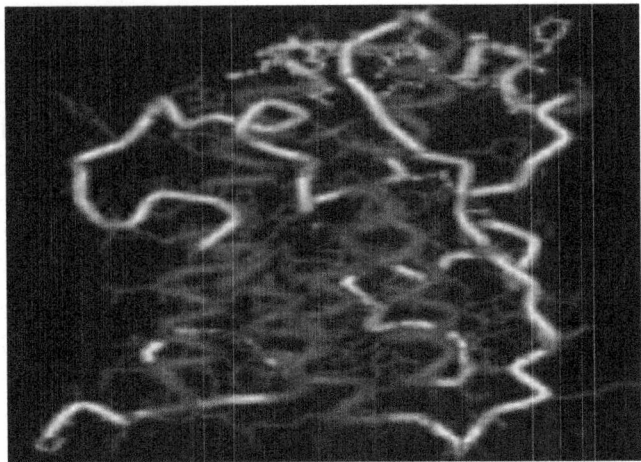

Fig. 11.2 Human growth hormone in its correct 22-kD-hGH form. Three-dimensional structure, generated from the protein data base SWISS PROT. Structural data supplied with the help of the program RasMol. The n-terminal amino acid (at the bottom left hand corner) are the disulphide bridges (and the sequence range missing on the 20 kDa hGH variant). The ranges with an α-Helix-structure are centrally located

or adjust T_4 substitutive therapy. Alcantara et al. (2006) demonstrated untreated GHD due to a homozygous GH releasing hormone receptor (GHRHR) mutation and heterozygous carriers of the same mutation have smaller thyroid volume than normal subjects, suggesting that GH has a permissive role in the growth of the thyroid gland (Fig. 11.2).

The Effects of Insulin on Anthropometry and Appearance

Athletes have been misguided by peer pressure and have strived to extrapolate the effects of the peptide hormone insulin, propagated by unsubstantiated myths, to their athletic performance. Such myths also pervade the health and fitness industry at an amateur level and have misled individuals into believing insulin may have a beneficial effect on cosmetic appearance. Hill and Milner (1985) have shown that insulin is a potent mitogen for many cell types in vitro. They concluded that insulin promotes the growth of selected tissues by a direct action. However, in the musculoskeletal system, the action is indirect, via the regulation of IGF-I release.

Sato et al. (1986) demonstrated that exogenous insulin caused an increase in glucose metabolism in athletes (measured by a euglycaemic insulin-clamp technique) and was significantly higher than controls. However, protein synthesis is thought not to be performed by insulin but by its regulation of insulin-like growth factor (IGF-I) and GH (Bennet et al. 1990). Its anabolic actions are believed to improve performance, by increasing protein synthesis (Kimball et al. 1994) and inhibiting protein catabolism and enhancing transport of selected amino acids in human skeletal muscle (Biolo et al. 1995). Hyper-aminoacidaemia specifically stimulates muscle protein synthesis and that even in the presence of hyper-aminoacidaemia insulin improves muscle protein balance, solely by inhibiting proteolysis. Hyper-aminoacidaemia combined with IGF-I enhances protein synthesis more than either alone (Fryburg et al. 1995).

It can be seen how the information that insulin treated diabetics are known to have increased LBM versus non-insulin-dependent diabetics can be misconceived (Sinha et al. 1996). The fact remains that insulin induces body weight gain by protecting lean mass, but also leads to fat accumulation in type 2 diabetes mellitus (Rigalleau et al. 1999). In addition to its role in regulating glucose metabolism, insulin increases amino acid transport into cells. Its stimulation of lipogenesis, and diminished lipolysis, was one of the reasons why bodybuilders and athletes would take rhGH in conjunction, to counteract this adverse effect, whilst optimizing protein synthesis. Insulin modulates transcription, altering the cell content of numerous (messenger-ribonucleic acids) mRNAs. It stimulates growth, DNA synthesis, and cell replication (Sonksen and Sonksen 2000; Sonksen 2001).

Prior to the availability of IGF-I, it was the inhibition of proteolysis that the "informed" athlete was interested in. Their belief was that administration of exogenous insulin, establishes an in-vivo hyper-insulinaemic clamp, would increase muscle glycogen, before and in the recovery stages of strenuous exercise. This was believed by the athlete to increase power, strength, and stamina, and therefore, assist recovery. Secondly, by inhibiting muscle protein breakdown and in conjunction with a high protein/high carbohydrate diet, insulin will have the action of increasing muscle bulk, potentially improving performance and appearance. There can be no doubt that exogenous insulin will not improve cosmetic appearance in athletes and that owing to its history of causing hypoglycaemia without supervision, its use can only be dangerous. It remains a mystery that it has maintained the status as a prescription-only medicine.

Metformin

Metformin has been a first-line treatment for type 2 diabetes mellitus for decades and is the most widely prescribed antidiabetic drug with normal kidney function, in particular, in the overweight (Dunn and Peters 1995). It is currently being prescribed to over 120 million people providing very interesting data. Metformin is an oral antidiabetic drug in the biguanide class. Internet forums suggest that Metformin is being used in the health and fitness industry and slimming clinics to aid weight loss and improve cosmetic appearance (http://www.redbookmag.com/health-wellness/advice/metformin-glucophage-weight-loss). It has been investigated where insulin resistance may be an important factor. Metformin works by suppressing glucose production by the liver. It lowers plasma concentrations of fasting insulin, total cholesterol and low density lipoprotein-cholesterol, free fatty acids, and tissue plasminogen activator antigen, a marker of endothelial damage (Charles and Eschwège 1999). In the clinical medicine management of poorly controlled type 2 diabetes mellitus, metformin is increasingly being used in combination with newer medications, exenatide (Byetta) or liraglutide (Victoza) (Scholz and Fleischmann 2014). They are glucagon-like protein 1 receptor agonists, which suppress appetite and are delivered by subcutaneous injection.

Metformin lowers glucose levels and is thought to increase insulin sensitivity, suppressing appetite, and calorie consumption. Exenatide or liraglutide delays the movement of food from the stomach into the small intestine, extending fullness and also suppressing appetite and calorie consumption. There will always be concerns re: injections of medication versus oral medication in the UK, the preference being oral medication. The molecular mechanism of metformin is believed to be inhibition of the mitochondrial respiratory chain (complex I), activation of AMP-activated protein kinase (AMPK), inhibition of glucagon-induced elevation of cyclic adenosine monophosphate (cAMP), and consequent activation of protein kinase A (PKA), inhibition of mitochondrial glycerophosphate dehydrogenase, and an effect on gut microbiota have been proposed as potential mechanisms. Activation of AMPK, an enzyme that plays an important role in insulin signalling, whole body energy balance, and the metabolism of glucose and fats were required for metformin's inhibitory effect on the production of glucose by liver cells. Activation of AMPK was required for an increase in the expression of small heterodimer partner, which in turn inhibited the expression of the hepatic gluconeogenic genes Phosphoenolpyruvate carboxykinase and glucose 6-phosphatase. Metformin and other biguanides may antagonize the action of glucagon, thus reducing fasting glucose levels. In addition to suppressing hepatic glucose production, metformin increases insulin sensitivity, enhances peripheral glucose uptake (by inducing the phosphorylation of GLUT4 enhancer factor), decreases insulin-induced suppression of fatty acid oxidation, and decreases absorption of glucose from the gastrointestinal tract. Increased peripheral use of glucose may be due to improved insulin binding to insulin receptors. AMPK probably also plays a role, as metformin administration increases AMPK activity in skeletal muscle. AMPK is known to cause GLUT4 deployment to the plasma membrane, resulting in insulin-independent glucose uptake. It is also believed to be associated with reduced risk of cancer (Luengo et al. 2014).

Metformin is now considered an old medication. Despite a systematic review in 2004, demonstrating that metformin was associated with decreased mortality after ten years in obese people with type 2 diabetes, there was no evidence to suggest that it decreased body fat and improved cosmesis (Avenell et al. 2004). The pharmaceutical companies are investigating the newer medications, such as glucagon-like protein 1 receptor agonists, which suppress appetite and comparing them to interventive surgery. Bariatric surgery is very effective for the management of morbid obesity, but there are always associated risks. Twelve months after bariatric surgery treatment versus liraglutide, the average weight loss was 38 kg in the bariatric surgery patients, versus 5 kg in medical treatment group. Glycaemic control improved in both groups but was greater in the bariatric surgery patients. The cardiovascular risk scores decreased in both groups, but remained higher in the medical treatment than in bariatric surgery patients. Of note, almost 60 % of patients on liraglutide met the target of glycated haemoglobin <7 % (53 mmol/ml) and lost ≥5 % of body weight (Cotugno et al. 2015). New data from the P3a SCALE Obesity and Pre-diabetes trial was presented at Obesity Week 2014, the 2nd Annual Congress of The American Society for Metabolic and Bariatric Surgery and The Obesity Society. In the liraglutide 3 mg group, 92 % of patients lost weight, in combination with diet and exercise, compared with 65 % on the placebo treatment in the 56-week study. Patients treated with liraglutide experienced weight loss of 9.2 % compared with a 3.5 % reduction in the placebo group. Patients who received liraglutide were found to experience improvements in quality of life scores too (http://www.ukmi.nhs.uk/applications/ndo/record_view_open.asp?newDrugID=4884). This data will go a long way to providing the new licence of the drug liraglutide in the management of weight loss in obesity in 2015, under the proprietary name Saxenda. Saxenda's use in sport as a performance and image-enhancing drug and its detection will remain to be elucidated. If it is perceived, however, that it is performance enhancing, it will be immediately included in the prohibited list.

Mechano Growth Factor (MGF)/ (IGF-1 Ec Peptide)

Mechano growth factor (MGF) has been identified and appears to be derived from the IGF-1 gene and has a unique C-terminal peptide (IGF-1 Ec peptide). It has a molecular weight of 2868 Da. After resistance exercise, which may cause disruption and damage to the myofibril cell membranes, the IGF-1 gene predominantly produces the IGF-1 splice variant IGF-1 Ec peptide (MGF) which activates muscle stem (satellite) cells or muscle progenitor cells that provide the extra nuclei required for muscle hypertrophy, repair and maintenance. The appearance of MGF also up-regulates new protein synthesis. After this initial splicing of IGF-1 into MGF, production then switches towards producing a systemic release of IGF-1 Ea from the liver, which also up-regulates protein synthesis. The expression of IGF-1 splice variants, over the course of the regeneration of muscle, following stress, is thought to be the primary anabolic mechanism by which the body repairs injuries or produces new muscle. Sarcopaenia (age related muscle atrophy) and dystrophic muscle appear to have an impaired ability to express MGF or refresh the satellite cell pool (Yang and Goldspink 2002). Muscle development must therefore be under the control of local growth factors because if a specific muscle is mechanically overloaded, as in resistant exercise, it is that muscle and not all the muscles that undergo hypertrophy.

Unlike mature IGF-1, the distinct E domain of MGF inhibits terminal differentiation whilst increasing myoblast proliferation. Blocking the IGF-1 receptor with a specific antibody indicates that the function of MGF E domain is mediated via a different receptor, providing localized tissue adaptation and suggesting why loss of muscle mass occurs in the elderly and in dystrophic muscle in which MGF production is markedly affected (Yang and Goldspink 2002). Such potential has attracted the attention of commercial companies claiming to be able to manufacture such peptide hormones for athletic abuse. MGF is available as an injectable peptide, and it has been shown that injecting it will increase local muscle growth (Goldspink 2005). The MGF peptide promises to be a potential treatment for the neuromuscular dystrophies. Its extrapolation into performance and image enhancement was considered within a very short period of time. The presence of a 'full-length MGF' provided by the Internet channels is freely available, with genuine associated scientific research articles also being provided explaining how their products work (http://www.peptidesciences.com/mgf). The provenance and safety of such products, however, would only be able to be verified by batch testing, which is not freely available. These products are not available in the NHS and would be considered by the authorities as counterfeit. MGF was considered undetectable in sport in doping analysis until recent research which has characterized a biotechnologically produced full-length MGF, using mass spectrometry, in doping controls (Thevis et al. 2014a, b). See Fig. 11.3 (IGF-1). MGF is a splice variant of IGF-I.

IGF-1 consists of 70 amino acids in a single chain with three intramolecular disulfide bridges. IGF-1 has a molecular weight of 7,649 daltons.

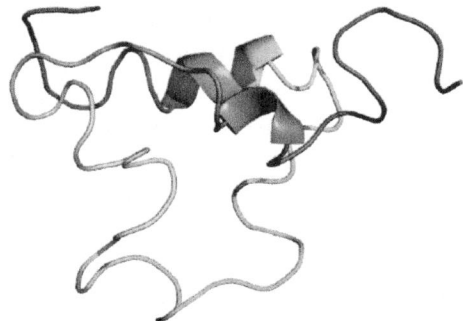

Fig. 11.3 Insulin-like growth factor (IGF-I)

A Myostatin Inhibitor (Follistatin)

Myostatin is a transforming growth factor-β (TGF-β) family member that plays an essential role in regulating skeletal muscle growth and associated body fat percentage. It acts as a negative regulator of skeletal muscle mass. Pharmacological agents capable of blocking myostatin activity may have applications for promoting muscle growth in human disease and reducing overall percentage of body fat. Follistatin, also known as activin-binding protein is a peptide hormone, in humans, encoded by the FST gene. Follistatin is an autocrine glycoprotein that is expressed in nearly all tissues. It is part of the inhibin-activin-follistatin axis and is produced by folliculostellate (FS) cells of the anterior pituitary. In the tissues activin has a strong role in cellular proliferation, thereby making follistatin the safeguard against uncontrolled cellular proliferation and also allowing it to function as an instrument of cellular differentiation. Both of these roles are vital in tissue rebuilding and repair. Follistatin, an antagonist to myostatin demonstrated that inhibition of myostatin, either by genetic elimination (knockout mice) or by increasing the amount of follistatin, resulted in greatly increased muscle mass (Lee and McPherron 2001). Obesity develops when energy intake exceeds energy expenditure, and is a major risk factor for the development of type 2 diabetes, dyslipidaemia, and subsequently cardiovascular disease. The imbalance between white adipose tissue (WAT) and brown adipose tissue (BAT) has been believed to be responsible for obesity and related metabolic diseases for over 30 years. Members of the TGF-β superfamily play an important role in regulating overall energy homeostasis by upregulation of brown adipocyte characteristics. Inactivation of TGF-β/Smad3/myostatin (Mst) signalling promotes browning of white adipocytes, increases mitochondrial biogenesis, and protects mice from diet-induced obesity. Follistatin has been shown to reduce insulin resistance, and the development of obesity and type 2 diabetes in mice (Singh et al. 2014). Naturally occurring myostatin gene mutations lead to a hypermuscular phenotype in humans (Schuelke et al. 2004). Eighteen months' administration of rhGH reduced myostatin levels in muscle of GHD hypopituitary adult patients and this was associated with an increase in LBM (Liu et al. 2003). This suggested that rhGH expressed its anabolic action by down-regulating myostatin. The application for treatment of not only genetic but also the hypokinetic diseases would appear to be very exciting, but human research is in its infancy. Despite being available through the Internet the websites specify that Follistatin is for research purposes and not for human consumption (http://www.peptidesciences.com/mgf). Inevitably, however, the performance and image enhancement industry will get wind of such information and attempt to exploit it. Then endocrinologists will either be assessing the consequences and applying the lessons learned to manage currently untreatable diseases or playing 'catch up' attempting to detect and ban it.

Conclusion

All drugs or medicines have side effects, which are exacerbated if the dosages taken are excessive. In the UK, the Internet has allowed the general populous to self-medicate by importation of medicines that were previously otherwise unavailable. Countries other than the UK have laws which allow exportation of such drugs and the UK laws allow their use, under the Medicines Act, 1968. There are minimal data on such unmonitored practices. However, it cannot be good for the health of the nation to continue in such a chaotic manner.

References

Alcantara, M. R., Salvatori, R., Alcantara, P. R., Nóbrega, L. M., Campos, V. S., Oliveira, E. C., et al. (2006). Thyroid morphology and function in adults with untreated isolated growth hormone deficiency. *The Journal of Clinical Endocrinology and Metabolism, 91*, 860–864.

Argetsinger, L. S., Campbell, G. S., Yang, X., Witthuhn, B. A., Silvennoinen, O., Ihle, J. N., et al. (1993). Identification of JAK2 as a growth hormone receptor-associated tyrosine kinase. *Cell, 74*, 237–244.

Avenell, A., Broom, J., Brown, T. J., Poobalan, A., Aucott, L., Stearns, S. C., et al. (2004). Systematic review of the long-term effects and economic consequences of treatments for obesity and implications for health improvement. *Health Technology Assessment, 8*, 1–182.

Baumann, G. (1991). Growth hormone heterogeneity: Genes, isohormones, variants, and binding proteins. *Endocrine Reviews, 12*, 424–449.

Bennet, W. M., Connacher, A. A., & Scrimgeour, C. M. (1990). Euglycaemic hyperinsulinaemia augments amino acid uptake by human leg tissues during hyperaminoacidaemia. *The American Journal of Physiology, 259*, 185–194.

Biolo, G., Fleming, R. Y. D., & Wolfe, R. D. (1995). Physiologic hyperinsulinaemia stimulates protein synthesis and enhances transport of selected amino acids in human skeletal muscle. *The Journal of Clinical Investigation, 95*, 811–819.

Boroujerdi, M. A., Umpleby, A. M., Jones, R. H., & Sonksen, P. H. (1995). A simulation model for glucose kinetics and estimates of glucose utilization rate in type I diabetic patients. *The American Journal of Physiology, 268*, 766–774.

Brown, R. J., Adams, J. J., Pelekanos, R. A., Wan, Y., McKinstry, W. J., Palethorpe, K., et al. (2005). Model for growth hormone receptor activation based on subunit rotation within a receptor dimer. *Nature Structural & Molecular Biology, 12*, 814–821.

Camacho-Hübner, C., Rose, S., Preece, M. A., Sleevi, M., Storr, H. L., Miraki-Moud, F., et al. (2006). Pharmacokinetic studies of recombinant human insulin-like growth factor I (rhIGF-I)/rhIGF-binding protein-3 complex administered to patients with growth hormone insensitivity syndrome. *Clinics in Endocrinology and Metabolism, 91*, 1246–1253.

Carroll, P. V., Christ, E. R., Bengtsson, B. A., Carlsson, L., Christiansen, J. S., Clemmons, D., et al. (1998). Growth hormone deficiency in adulthood and the effects of growth hormone replacement: A review. Growth Hormone

Research Society Scientific Committee. *The Journal of Clinical Endocrinology and Metabolism, 83*, 382–395.

Charles, M. A., & Eschwège, E. (1999). Prevention of type 2 diabetes: Role of metformin. *Drugs and Supplements, 1*, 71–73 discussion 75–82.

Cotugno, M., Nosso, G., Saldalamacchia, G., Vitagliano, G., Griffo, E., Lupoli, R., et al. (2015). Clinical efficacy of bariatric surgery versus liraglutide in patients with type 2 diabetes and severe obesity: A 12-month retrospective evaluation. *Acta Diabetologica, 52*(2), 331–336.

Crist, D. M., Peake, G. T., Egan, P. A., & Waters, D. L. (1988). Body composition response to exogenous GH during training in highly conditioned adults. *Journal of Applied Physiology, 65*, 579–584.

Dawson, R. T. (2001). Drugs in sport. The role of the physician. *Journal of Endocrinology, 170*, 55–61.

Duchaine, D. (1983). *Underground steroid handbook* (1st ed.p. 84). California: HLR Technical Books.

Dunn, C. J., & Peters, D. H. (1995). Metformin. A review of its pharmacological properties and therapeutic use in non-insulin-dependent diabetes mellitus. *Drugs, 49*, 721–749.

Ehrnborg, C., Ellegard, L., Bosaeus, I., Bengtsson, B. A., & Rosen, T. (2005). Supraphysiological growth hormone: Less fat, more extracellular fluid but uncertain effects on muscles in healthy, active young adults. *Clinical Endocrinology, 62*, 449–457.

Elbornsson, M., Götherström, G., Bosæus, I., Bengtsson, B. Å., Johannsson, G., & Svensson, J. (2013). Fifteen years of GH replacement improves body composition and cardiovascular risk factors. *European Journal of Endocrinology, 15*, 745–753.

Erotokritou-Mulligan, I., Eryl Bassett, E., Cowan, D. A., Bartlett, C., Milward, P., Sartorio, A., et al. (2010). The use of growth hormone (GH)-dependent markers in the detection of GH abuse in sport: Physiological intra-individual variation of IGF-I, type 3 pro-collagen (P-III-P) and the GH-2000 detection score. *Clinical Endocrinology, 72*, 520–526.

Erotokritou-Mulligan, I., Holt, R. I., & Sönksen, P. H. (2011). Growth hormone doping: A review. *Open Access Journal of Sports Medicine, 2*, 99–111.

Evans, P. J., & Lynch, R. M. (2003). Insulin as a drug of abuse in body building. *British Journal of Sports Medicine, 37*, 356–357.

Fryburg, D. A., Jahn, L. A., Hill, S. A., Oliveras, D. M., & Barrett, E. J. (1995). Insulin and Insulin-like Growth Factor-I enhance human skeletal muscle protein anabolism during hyperaminoacidaemia by different mechanisms. *The Journal of Clinical Investigation, 96*, 1722–1729.

Goeddel, D. V., Heyneker, H. L., Hozumi, T., Arentzen, R., Itakura, K., Yansura, D. G., et al. (1979). Direct expression in *Escherichia coli* of a DNA sequence coding for human growth hormone. *Nature, 281*, 544–548.

Goldspink, G. (2005). Research on mechano growth factor: Its potential for optimising physical training as well as misuse in doping. *British Journal of Sports Medicine, 39*, 787–788.

Grace, F. M., Baker, J. S., & Davies, B. (2001). Anabolic androgenic steroid (AAS) use in recreational gym users—A regional sample of the Mid-Glamorgan area. *Journal of Substance Use, 12*, 145–153.

Graham, M. R., Baker, J. S., & Davies, B. (2006). "Steroid" and prescription medicine abuse in the health and fitness community; A regional study. *European Journal of Internal Medicine, 17*, 479–484.

Graham, M. R., Baker, J. S., Evans, P., Hullin, D., Thomas, N. E., & Davies, B. (2009). Potential benefits of recombinant human growth hormone (rhGH) to athletes. *Growth Hormone & IGF Research, 19*, 300–307.

Graham, M. R., Evans, P., Davies, B., & Baker, J. S. (2008). AAS, growth hormone, and insulin abuse: Psychological and neuroendocrine effects. *Therapeutics and Clinical Risk Management, 4*, 587–597.

Greig, C. A., Hameed, M., Young, A., Goldspink, G., & Noble, B. (2006). Skeletal muscle IGF-I isoform expression in healthy women after isometric exercise. *Growth Hormone & IGF Research, 16*, 373–376.

Grunfeld, C., Sherman, B. M., & Cavalieri, R. R. (1988). The acute effects of human growth hormone administration on thyroid function in normal men. *The Journal of Clinical Endocrinology and Metabolism, 67*, 1111–1114.

Guler, H. P., Zapf, J., Schmid, C., & Froesch, E. R. (1989). Insulin-like growth factors I and II in healthy man estimations of half-lives and production rates. *Acta Endocrinologica, 121*, 753–758.

Healy, M. L., Gibney, J., Pentecost, C., Croos, P., Russell-Jones, D. L., Sönksen, P. H., et al. (2006). Effects of high-dose growth hormone on glucose and glycerol metabolism at rest and during exercise in endurance-trained athletes. *The Journal of Clinical Endocrinology and Metabolism, 9*, 320–327.

Healy, M. L., Gibney, J., Russell-Jones, D. L., Pentecost, C., Croos, P., Sönksen, P. H., et al. (2003). High dose growth hormone exerts an anabolic effect at rest and during exercise in endurance-trained athletes. *The Journal of Clinical Endocrinology and Metabolism, 11*, 5221–5226.

Hill, D. J., & Milner, R. D. G. (1985). Insulin as a growth factor. *Paediatric Research, 19*, 879–886.

Holt, R. I. (2013). Detecting growth hormone misuse in athletes. *Indian Journal of Endocrinology Metabolism, 17*, 18–22.
Holt, R. I., & Sönksen, P. H. (2008). Growth hormone, IGF-I and insulin and their abuse in sport. *British Journal of Pharmacology, 154*, 542–556.
http://www.tas-cas.org/d2wfiles/document/6633/5048/0/256620FINAL20Award20_internet_.pdf. Accessed 1 December 2014.
http://www.paralympic.org/press-release/latest-testing-methods-result-suspension-two-russian-powerlifters-anti-doping. Accessed 1 December 2014.
http://www.ukad.org.uk/news/article/uk-research-leads-to-new-growth-hormone-test. Accessed 1 December 2014.
http://www.redbookmag.com/health-wellness/advice/metformin-glucophage-weight-loss. Accessed 1 December 2014.
http://www.ukmi.nhs.uk/applications/ndo/record_view_open.asp?newDrugID=4884. Accessed 1 December 2014.
http://www.peptidesciences.com/mgf. Accessed 8 December 2014.
Iranmanesh, A., Lizarralde, G., & Velduis, J. D. (1991). Age and relative adiposity are specific negative determinants of the frequency and amplitude of growth hormone secretory bursts and the half-life of endogenous GH in healthy men. *The Journal of Clinical Endocrinology and Metabolism, 73*, 1081–1088.
Johannsson, G., Grimby, G., Sunnerhagen, K. S., & Bengtsson, B. A. (1997). Two years of growth hormone (GH) treatment increases isometric and isokinetic muscle strength in GH-deficient adults. *The Journal of Clinical Endocrinology and Metabolism, 82*, 2877–2884.
Kemp, S. F. (2007). Mecasermin rinfabate. *Drugs Today, 43*, 149–155.
Kimball, S. R., Vary, T. C., & Jefferson, L. S. (1994). Regulation of protein synthesis by insulin. *Annual Review of Physiology, 56*, 321–348.
Kojima, M., Hosoda, H., Date, Y., Nakazato, M., Matsuo, H., & Kangawa, K. (1999). Ghrelin is a growth-hormone-releasing acylated peptide from stomach. *Nature, 9*, 656–660.
Konrad, C., Schupfer, G., Wietlisbach, M., & Gerber, H. (1998). Insulin as an anabolic: Hypoglycaemia in the bodybuilding world. *Anaesthesiol Intensivmed Schmerzther, 33*, 461–463.
Lange, K. H., Andersen, J. L., Beyer, N., Isaksson, F., Larsson, B., Rasmussen, M. H., et al. (2002). GH admin changes myosin heavy chain isoforms in skeletal muscle but does not augment muscle strength or hypertrophy, either

alone or combined with resistance exercise training in healthy elderly men. *The Journal of Clinical Endocrinology and Metabolism, 87*, 513–523.

Lee, S. J., & McPherron, A. C. (2001). Regulation of myostatin activity and muscle growth. *Proceedings of the National Academy of Sciences of the United States of America, 98*, 9306–9311.

Le Roith, D., Scavo, L., & Butler, A. (2001). What is the role of circulating IGF-I? *Trends in Endocrinology and Metabolism, 12*, 48–52.

Li, C. H., & Papkoff, H. (1956). Preparation and properties of growth hormone from human and monkey pituitary glands. *Science, 124*, 1293–1294.

Liu, W., Thomas, S. G., Asa, S. L., Gonzalez-Cadavid, N., Bhasin, S., & Ezzat, S. (2003). Myostatin is a skeletal muscle target of growth hormone anabolic action. *The Journal of Clinical Endocrinology and Metabolism, 88*, 5490–5496.

Luengo, A., Sullivan, L. B., & Heiden, M. G. (2014). Understanding the complexity of metformin action: Limiting mitochondrial respiration to improve cancer therapy. *BMC Biology, 12*, 82.

Mauras, N., Attie, K. M., Reiter, E. O., Saenger, P., & Baptista, J. (2000). High dose recombinant human growth hormone (GH) treatment of GH-deficient patients in puberty increases near-final height: A randomized, multicenter trial. Genentech, Inc., Cooperative Study Group. *The Journal of Clinical Endocrinology and Metabolism, 85*, 3653–3660.

Mauras, N., & Haymond, M. W. (2005). Are the metabolic effects of GH and IGF-I separable. *Growth Hormone & IGF Research, 15*, 19–27.

Melmed, S. (2006). Medical progress: Acromegaly. *The New England Journal of Medicine, 14*, 2558–2573.

Milani, D., Carmichael, J. D., Welkowitz, J., Ferris, S., Reitz, R. E., Danoff, A., et al. (2004). Variability and reliability of single serum IGF-I measurements: Impact on determining predictability of risk ratios in disease development. *The Journal of Clinical Endocrinology and Metabolism, 89*, 2271–2274.

O'Reilly, K. E., Rojo, F., She, Q. B., Solit, D., Mills, G. B., Smith, D., et al. (2006). mTOR inhibition induces upstream receptor tyrosine kinase signaling and activates Akt. *Cancer Research, 66*, 1500–1508.

Papadakis, M. A., Grady, D., Black, D., Tierney, M. J., Gooding, G. A., Schambelan, M., et al. (1996). Growth hormone replacement in healthy older men improves body composition but not functional ability. *Annals of Internal Medicine, 124*, 708–716.

Porretti, S., Giavoli, C., Ronchi, C., Lombardi, G., Zaccaria, M., Valle, D., et al. (2002). Recombinant human GH replacement therapy and thyroid function in a large group of adult GH-deficient patients: When does L-T(4) therapy become mandatory? *The Journal of Clinical Endocrinology and Metabolism, 87*, 2042–2045.

Portes, E. S., Oliveira, J. H., MacCagnan, P., & Abucham, J. (2000). Changes in serum thyroid hormones levels and their mechanisms during long-term growth hormone (GH) replacement therapy in GH deficient children. *Clinical Endocrinology, 53*, 183–189.

Powrie, J. K., Bassett, E. E., Rosen, T., Jørgensen, J. O., Napoli, R., Sacca, L., et al. (2007). Detection of growth hormone abuse in sport. On behalf of the GH-2000 Project study group. *Growth Hormone & IGF Research, 17*, 220–226.

Rigalleau, V., Delafaye, C., Baillet, L., Vergnot, V., Brunou, P., Gatta, B., et al. (1999). Composition of insulin-induced body weight gain in diabetic patients: A bio-impedance study. *Diabetes & Metabolism, 4*, 321–328.

Rinderknecht, E., & Humbel, R. E. (1978). The amino acid sequence of human insulin-like growth factor I and its structural homology with proinsulin. *The Journal of Biological Chemistry, 253*, 2769–2776.

Rudman, D., Feller, A. G., Cohn, L., Shetty, K. R., Rudman, I. W., & Draper, M. W. (1991). Effect of human growth hormone on body composition in elderly men. *Hormone Research, 36*, 73–81.

Salomon, F., Cuneo, R. C., Hesp, R., & Sonksen, P. H. (1989). The effects of treatment with recombinant human growth hormone on body composition and metabolism in adults with growth hormone deficiency. *The New England Journal of Medicine, 321*, 1797–1803.

Sato, Y., Hayamizu, S., Yamamoto, C., Ohkuwa, Y., Yamanouchi, K., & Sakamoto, N. (1986). Improved insulin sensitivity in carbohydrate and lipid metabolism after physical training. *International Journal of Sports Medicine, 7*, 307–310.

Schafer, E. (1916). *The endocrine organs*. London: Longman, Green & Co.

Scholz, G. H., & Fleischmann, H. (2014). Basal insulin combined incretin mimetic therapy with glucagon-like protein 1 receptor agonists as an upcoming option in the treatment of type 2 diabetes: A practical guide to decision making. *Therapeutic Advances in Endocrinology and Metabolism, 5*, 95–123 Review.

Schuelke, M., Wagner, K. R., Stolz, L. E., Hubner, C., Riebel, T., Komen, W., et al. (2004). Myostatin mutation associated with gross muscle hypertrophy in a child. *The New England Journal of Medicine, 350*, 2682–2688.

Sigurjonsdottir, H. A., Koranyi, J., Axelson, M., Bengtsson, B. A., & Johannsson, G. (2006). GH effect on enzyme activity of 11betaHSD in abdominal obesity is dependent on treatment duration. *European Journal of Endocrinology, 154*, 69–74.

Singh, R., Braga, M., & Pervin, S. (2014). Regulation of brown adipocyte metabolism by myostatin/follistatin signaling. Review. *Frontiers in Cell Developmental Biology, 2*, 60.

Sinha, A., Formica, C., Tsalamandris, C., Panagiotopoulos, S., Hendrich, E., DeLuise, M., et al. (1996). Effects of insulin on body composition in patients with insulin-dependent and non-insulin-dependent diabetes. *Diabetic Medicine, 13*, 40–46.

Sonksen, P. H. (2001). Insulin, growth hormone and sport. *Journal of Endocrinology, 170*, 13–25.

Sonksen, P. H., & Sonksen, J. (2000). Insulin: Understanding its action in health and disease. *British Journal of Anaesthesia, 85*, 69–79.

Thevis, M., Thomas, A., Delahaut, P., Bosseloir, A., & Schanzer, W. (2006). Doping control analysis of intact rapid-acting insulin analogues in human urine by liquid chromatography-tandem mass spectro-metry. *Analytical Chemistry, 78*, 1897–1903.

Thevis, M., Thomas, A., Geyer, H., & Schänzer, W. (2014a). Mass spectrometric characterization of a biotechnologically produced full-length mechano growth factor (MGF) relevant for doping controls. *Growth Hormone & IGF Research, 24*, 276–280.

Thevis, M., Thomas, A., & Schänzer, W. (2014b). Detecting peptidic drugs, drug candidates and analogs in sports doping: Current status and future directions. *Expert Review of Proteomics, 11*, 663–673.

Thomas, A., Thevis, M., Delahaut, P., Bosseloir, A., & Schanzer, W. (2007). Mass spectrometric identification of degradation products of insulin and its long-acting analogues in human urine for doping control purposes. *Analytical Chemistry, 79*, 2518–2524.

Thomas, S. H. L., Wisher, M. H., Brandenburg, D., & Sonksen, P. H. (1979). Insulin action on adipocytes. Evidence that the anti-lipolytic and lipogenic effects of insulin are medicated by the same receptor. *The Biochemical Journal, 184*, 355–360.

Wallace, J. D., Cuneo, R. C., Baxter, R., Orskov, H., Keay, N., Pentecost, C., et al. (1999). Responses of the growth hormone (GH) and insulin-like growth factor axis to exercise, GH administration and GH withdrawal in trained adult males: A potential test for GH abuse in sport. *The Journal of Clinical Endocrinology and Metabolism, 84,* 3591–3601.

Wu, Z., Bidlingmaier, M., Dall, R., & Strasburger, C. J. (1999). Detection of doping with human growth hormone. *Lancet, 353,* 895.

Wyatt, D. T., Gesundheit, N., & Sherman, B. (1998). Changes in thyroid hormone levels during growth hormone therapy in initially euthyroid patients: Lack of need for thyroxine supplementation. *The Journal of Clinical Endocrinology and Metabolism, 83,* 3493–3497.

Yang, S. Y., & Goldspink, G. (2002). Different roles of the IGF-I Ec peptide (MGF) and mature IGF-I in myoblast proliferation and differentiation. *FEBS Letters, 522,* 156–160.

Yarasheki, K. E., Zachwieja, J. J., Campbell, J. A., & Bier, D. M. (1995). Effect of growth hormone and resistance exercise on muscle growth and strength in older men. *The American Journal of Physiology, 268,* 268–276.

Afterword: Toward an Inclusive, Multi-Disciplinary Approach to Understanding Substance Use for Appearance Purposes

Brendan Gough, Sarah Grogan, and Matthew Hall

With this edited collection, we have tried to provide the latest insights into a phenomenon which is attracting more and more attention from researchers, health professionals, and the media in general—the use of chemical substances to enhance appearance. This is a developing field which is producing insights from a range of disciplinary perspectives, with concepts deployed from sociology, social and health psychology, psychiatry, and sports science, as featured within this book. We also note diverse research methods and studies, from experimental designs and analysis of chemical side effects of various substances to

---

B. Gough
School of Social, Psychological and Communication Sciences, Leeds Beckett University, Calverly Building [Rm 919], City Campus, LS1 9HE, Leeds, UK

S. Grogan
Department of Psychology, Manchester Metropolitan University, 53 Bonsall Street, M15 6GX, Manchester, UK

M. Hall
Associate Academic, University of Derby, Department of Psychology, Kedleston Road, Derby DE22 1GB, UK

© The Editor(s) (if applicable) and The Author(s) 2016
M. Hall et al. (eds.), *Chemically Modified Bodies*,
DOI 10.1057/978-1-137-53535-1

qualitative interviews and examination of media materials. What unites the chapters is a concern that many (mainly young) people are risking their health through recourse to chemicals in different guises in order to attain appearance-related goals such as weight loss or muscle inflation. All substances covered in this book are linked to serious side effects when taken inappropriately or in high doses, and the fact that many such substances can now be readily purchased online, without medical oversight, underlines the need for greater understanding and intervention in this field.

The majority of chapters focus on adolescents and young adults, reflecting the body image literature more generally, but in so doing rely heavily on samples of college students, as many authors note. This spotlight on younger people is clearly important, generating valuable insights into risky body practices and motivations which can then inform health promotion initiatives. But as the field grows it is also important to consider diverse samples and settings, including those young people who are marginalized by neighborhood, ethnicity, education, or employment status. At the same time, we must remember that body image issues and risky practices are not the preserve of young people alone. Apart from the area of weight management, body image research has not focused much on people aged 30 and above. However, there is evidence that older women and men may have similar levels of body dissatisfaction to younger people (Grogan 2012), and that older people may be sensitive to body image issues associated with aging, although this work has tended to focus on white women (Midarsky and Nitzberg 2008). A recent study by Gough et al. (2015), however, showed that overweight men, including some in their 60s, reported high levels of body dissatisfaction, while recent age-appearance facial morphing work with men (Flett et al. 2015; Grogan and Loosemore 2015; Williams et al. 2013) has highlighted that exposure to personalized face aging images caused young men to reflect on quitting smoking and to use sunscreen when in the sun, in order to reduce possible aging effects on their skin. As yet we are not aware of any research which investigates the use of substances by older people designed to enhance appearance.

Gender also appears as a key theme within this book and within body image literature more generally. It is now well established that boys and men as well as girls and women experience a range of body image issues, with a lean-but-muscular norm for males and a slim-but-curvaceous norm for females. The chapters in this book document trends in the deployment of specific substances for weight loss and greater muscularity, but there is more scope for examining substance use for other body projects, such as hair restoration and penis enlargement for men, or body hair removal and buttock implants for women. For example, Langdridge et al. (2013) highlight the wealth of online options for men seeking to extend penis size, but we know little about those men who pursue these options. While body projects and practices continue to largely reflect gendered norms, we must be careful not to reproduce stereotypes, to examine gender 'transgressions' such as women invested in muscularity and men diagnosed with eating disorders, and to study body image phenomena with transgender groups, including substance use. Clearly a minority of women desire a highly muscled appearance and will engage in anabolic steroid use to enable them to attain these high levels of muscle, possibly shifting their body-shape ideals to a more muscular figure, and their primary social reference group to those within the body building community (Grogan et al. 2004, 2006), and some men are highly invested in weight loss to try to attain a slender body (Morgan and Arcelus 2009). We must not presume that all women want to be thin and all men muscular, or even that gender is the most important factor in a given individual's embodied motivations.

Greater collaboration between disciplines is required for the field to advance further. Just as a greater understanding of the chemical and health effects of substances is needed, so too are further insights into the accounts provided by users about their motivations and desires, as well as (critical) consideration of the global and local contexts which conspire to present embodied risk-taking as an enticing option. In presenting diverse perspectives, studies, and concepts, this book marks an opening up of the field—a foundation on which we hope that researchers interested in body projects, consumption, and health will build.

References

Flett, K., Grogan, S., Clark-Carter, D., Gough, B., & Conner M. (2015). Male smokers' experiences of an appearance-focused facial-ageing intervention. *Journal of Health Psychology*. doi: 10.1177/1359105315603477.

Gough, B., Seymour-Smith, S., & Matthews, C. R. (2015). Body dissatisfaction, appearance investment and wellbeing: How older obese men orient to "aesthetic health". *Psychology of Men & Masculinity*.

Grogan, S. (2012). Body image development in adulthood. In T. F. Cash & L. Smolak (Ed.), *Body image: A handbook of science, practice, and prevention* (pp. 93–100). New York: Guilford Press.

Grogan, S., Evans, R., Wright, S., & Hunter, G. (2004). Femininity and muscularity: Accounts of seven women body builders. *Journal of Gender Studies*, 13, 1, 57–71.

Grogan, S., Shepherd, S., Evans, R., Wright, S., & Hunter, G. (2006). Body builders experiences of anabolic steroid use: In-depth interviews with men and women body builders. *Psychology and Health*, 11, 845–856.

Langdridge, D., Flowers, P., Gough, B., & Holliday, R. (2013). On the biomedicalisation of the penis: The commodification of function and aesthetics. *International Journal of Men's Health*, 12(2): 121–137.

Loosemore, E., & Grogan, S. (2015). Men's accounts of reactions to two sources of information on negative effects of UV exposure: Facial morphing and a health promotion fact sheet. *International Journal of Men's Health*. doi: 10.3149/jmh.1402.183.

Midlarsky, E., & Nitzburg, G. (2008). Eating disorders in middle-aged women. *Journal of General Psychology*, 135, 393–408.

Morgan, J. F., & Arcelus, J. (2009). Body image in gay and straight men: A qualitative study. *Eating Disorders Review*, 17, 435–443.

Williams, A., Grogan, S., Buckley, E., & Clark-Carter, D. (2013). Men's experiences of an appearance-focussed facial-ageing sun protection intervention: A qualitative study. *Body Image: An International Journal of Research*, 10, 263–266.

Index

A
ADHD medications
  pharmacology of, 151–3
  for weight loss, off-label use of, 153–5
Adolescent Experience Questionnaire, 17–18
advertising of nutritional/sports supplements, 93–106
  body dissatisfaction and, 94–6
  body image and, 94–6
  enhancement of, 96–8
  enhancement with health, merging, 98–102
  as forestate of future, 105–6
  as mirror to twenty-first century health, 102–5
aerobic exercise, and eating disorder, 32
age, and drug use, 18–19

amino acids, 62–3
AMP-activated protein kinase (AMPK), 217
amphetamines
  for ADHD, 152
  for weight loss, 56–7
anabolic-androgenic steroids (AAS), 55–6
  for muscle dysmorphia, 38–46
  perceived benefits of, 38–41
  and psychological addiction, 41–2
anabolic steroids, and muscularity, 6
anorexia nervosa (AN)
  caffeine use and, 85, 86
anthropometry
  growth hormone effects on, 210
  insulin effects on, 214–16
anti-obesity medications, 173–94
  clenbuterol, 177, 187–9
  dinitrophenol, 190–1

anti-obesity medications (*cont.*)
  ephedrine, 177, 181–4
  fenfluramine/phentermine, 178, 191
  future research of, 193–4
  levothyroxine, 186–7
  lorcaserin, 178, 191–2
  orlistat, 177, 179–81
  phentermine/topiramate, 177
  phenylpropanolamine, 178
  rimonabant, 178, 193–4
  sibutramine, 177, 189–91
  tetraiodothyronine, 177, 184–7
  topiramate, 192
  triiodothyronine, 177, 184–7
anxiety disorders, 35
appearance-and performance-enhancing drugs (APEDs), 53–4
  prevalence of, 14–16
  risk factors of, 16–25
appearance enhancement, defining and outlining drug use for, 53–5
appearance investment, 53
appearance work, 52–3
Athletes Training and Learning to Avoid Steroids (ATLAS) program, 68–9
atomoxetine, for weight loss, 153

B
binge eating disorder (BED)
  caffeine use and, 85
bodybuilders, synthol used by, 127–43
  credibility, 138–43
  data analysis, 131–2
  data collection, 129–30
  ethics of, 130–1
  legitimation, 133–4
  results, 132
  support, 134–7
bodybuilding, and muscle dysmorphia, 36–7, 41–2
body dissatisfaction, 19, 68, 69, 159, 232
  adolescent girls, 52
  and advertising, 94–6
  eating disorders and, 163–4
  muscle dysmorphia and, 32, 35, 37, 43, 44
  smoking and, 112–15, 119
body dysmorphic disorder (BDD), 33
  diagnostic criteria for, 34, 36
body image
  and advertising, 94–6
  attitudinal, 4
  boys, 13–25
  defined, 4
  drug use and, 3–5
  male adolescents, 13–25
  smoking and, 113–16
body mass index (BMI), 18, 81, 112
  classification of, 176, 179–80
body satisfaction, 5, 43, 69
  appearance investment and, 53
  smoking and, 113, 114
body weight, 24, 52, 174, 193, 215
  smoking and, 112–13
boys, use of supplements and drugs to change body image and appearance among, 13–25
  prevalence of, 14–16
  risk factors of, 16–25

types of, 14–16
bulimia nervosa (BN)
    caffeine use and, 85, 86

C
caffeine, 97
    abuse/misuse, *See* caffeine abuse/
        misuse
    mechanism of action, 79–80
    use, *See* caffeine use
    and weight loss, 16
    weight loss using, 5
caffeine abuse/misuse
    in normal populations, 81–3
    potential of, 80–1
caffeine use
    and eating disorders, 84–6
    and psychiatric disorders, 83–4
cigarette smoking, *See* smoking
clenbuterol
    for obesity, 177, 187–9
    for weight loss, 5
cocaine, for weight loss, 56–7
comorbid psychological disorders, 35
creatine, 62–3
cultural background, and drug use,
    20–1

D
dextroamphetamine, for ADHD,
    152
dextroamphetamine-amphetamine
    salts (Adderall), 152, 162
    for ADHD, 16, 151, 153
diet pills
    and weight loss, 15
    for weight loss, 5, 57–9

dinitrophenol (DNP), 190–1
discourse analysis, 131
disordered eating
    and weight control behaviours,
        163–4
    See also eating disorders (ED)
diuretics, for weight loss, 15, 58, 59,
    66, 86, 130, 191

E
eating disorders (ED)
    aerobic exercise and, 32
    caffeine use and, 84–7
e-cigarettes, 122
    See also smoking
ecstasy, for weight loss, 56–7
energy drinks, 97
enhancement
    with health, merging, 98–102
    performance, 97
    of sports and nutritional
        supplements, 96–8
Ephedra sinica (Ma Huang), 182
ephedrine, 83, 130
    alkaloids, for obesity, 177
    mechanism of action, 181–3
    recreational Use of, 183–4
    for weight loss, 5
exenatide (Byetta), 216
exercise prescription, 31

F
facial ageing, and smoking,
    116–19
female adolescents, drug use to
    change appearance in,
    51–70

female adolescents (*cont.*)
  amphetamines, 56–7
  anabolic-androgenic steroids, 55–6
  cigarette smoking, 60–2
  cocaine, 56–7
  defining and outlining, 53–5
  diet pills, 57–9
  ecstasy, 56–7
  health education theory for school-based prevention programs, use of, 67–9
  implications for school-based education, 65–7
  laxatives, 57–9
  nutritional supplements, 62–3
  slimming pills, 57–9
  stimulant drugs, 56–7
  tanning products, 64–5
fenfluramine/phentermine (Fen-Phen), for obesity, 178, 191
follistatin, 220–1
free fatty acid (FFA), 180, 209, 210

G

Gatorade, and muscularity, 15
gender-role stereotypes, drug use and, 25
girls, drug use to change appearance in, 51–70
  amphetamines, 56–7
  anabolic-androgenic steroids, 55–6
  cigarette smoking, 60–2
  cocaine, 56–7
  culture of, 51–3
  defining and outlining, 53–5
  diet pills, 57–9
  ecstasy, 56–7
  health education theory for school-based prevention programs, use of, 67–9
  implications for school-based education, 65–7
  laxatives, 57–9
  nutritional supplements, 62–3
  slimming pills, 57–9
  stimulant drugs, 56–7
  tanning products, 64–5
glucose transporters (GLUTs), 209, 210, 217
growth hormone
  effects in healthy individuals, 211–12
  effects on anthropometry, 210
  effects on thyroid function, 212–14
  human, 201
  and muscularity, 6
  physiology of, 205–8
  recombinant human growth, 201–2
  United Kingdom law and ethical consideration, 205
growth hormone releasing hormone (GHRH), 206

H

Health Belief Model, 67
health education theory, for school-based prevention programs, 67–9
human growth hormone (hGH), 201
  recombinant, 201–2, 212
hypothyroidism, 186

I

IGF-1 Ec peptide, 218–19
illicit drug use, during adolescence, 163
insulin
    effects on anthropometry and appearance, 214–16
    ethical consideration for, 205
    physiology of, 209–10
insulin-like growth factor-1 (IGF-1), 203–4, 220
    effects in healthy individuals, 211–12
    physiology of, 105–8
    United Kingdom law and ethical consideration, 205
insulin-like growth factor-2 (IGF-2), 203
insulin-like growth factor 1 receptor (IGF1R), 207

J

Janus kinase 2 (JAK2) protein, 206

L

laxatives, for weight loss, 15, 54, 55, 57–9, 60, 86, 157
leptin, 193
levothyroxine, abuse of, 186–7
liraglutide (Victoza), 216, 218
lisdexamfetamine
    for ADHD, 152–3
    for weight loss, 154
lorcaserin, for obesity, 178, 191–2

M

major depressive disorder, 35
male adolescents, use of supplements and drugs to change body image and appearance among, 13–25
    prevalence of, 14–16
    risk factors of, 16–25
    types of, 14–16
mechano growth factor (MGF), 207, 218–19
media exposure, drug use and, 19
Medicines Act, 1968, 205
metabolic clearance rate (MCR), 209, 210
metformin, 216–18
    ethical consideration for, 205
methamphetamine, for weight loss, 16, 24
methylenedioxymethamphetamine, 83
methylphenidate
    for ADHD, 152
    for weight loss, 153, 154
Misuse of Drugs Act, 1971, 205
muscle dysmorphia (MD), 33
    anaboilc steroids and, 6
    behavioural characteristics of, 36
    bodybuilding/weightlifting and, 36–7, 41–2
    diagnostic criteria for, 34–6
    performance-enhancing drugs and, 38–43
    treatment for, 44–6
muscularity, drug use and, 6, 14, 17, 19–23, 32, 43, 45, 46, 55
myostatin, 207, 220–1

N

negative affect, 23, 24, 115
non-medical use of prescription drugs (NMUPD), 149–50
non-medical use of prescription stimulants (NMUPS), 150–1
   during adolescence, use of, 163
   in college and non-college students, 161–2
   current research, limitations of, 161
   demographics of, 160–1
   as focal point, 156–9
   future directions of, 161, 164–5
   and stigma, 159–60
   for weight loss, 155–61, 162–3
N-terminal propeptide of type III procollagen (P-III-P), 202
nutritional supplements, advertising of, 93–106
   body dissatisfaction and, 94–6
   body image and, 94–6
   enhancement of, 96–8
   enhancement with health, merging, 98–102
   as foretaste of future, 105–6
   as mirror to twenty-first century health, 102–5
nutritional supplements, for weight loss, 62–3

O

obsessive-compulsive disorder (OCD), 35
opposite-gender peers-adolescent relationship, 24
orlistat (Xenical)
   mechanism of action, 180–1
   for obesity, 177, 179–80
   for weight loss, 5, 7, 190

P

parent-adolescent relationship, 24
phentermine/topiramate, for obesity, 178
phenylpropanolamine
   and haemorrhagic stroke, 191
   for obesity, 178
Powerade, and muscularity, 15
prescription drugs, non-medical use of, *See* non-medical use of prescription drugs (NMUPD)
prescription stimulants, non-medical use of, *See* non-medical use of prescription stimulants (NMUPS)
Prophet of Pit-1 (PROP1), 205
protein
   powder/supplements, 15, 24, 36, 62, 63, 130
   synthesis, 203, 215, 219
psychiatric disorders, caffeine use and, 83–4
psychological addiction, anabolic-androgenic steroids and, 41–2
pubertal development, drug use and, 18–19

R

recombinant human growth hormone (rhGH), 201–2
   dosage effects of, 212

for weight loss, 5
reverse anorexia, *See* muscle dysmorphia (MD)
rimonabant, for obesity, 178, 193–4
risk-taking behaviours
  boys, 22–3
  male adolescents, 22–3
Ritalin, for ADHD, 16, 151, 152, 162

S

school-based education
  drug and substance use to change appearance, implications of, 65–7
school-based prevention programs, health education theory for, 67–9
self-efficacy, 68, 87, 120
self-esteem, 16, 22–4, 31, 35–6, 45, 46, 52, 68, 82, 87, 115, 119, 157
serum biological passport analysis, 202–3
sibutramine, for obesity, 83, 176, 189–91
signal transducers and activators of transcription (STAT) proteins, 206
silica tablets, 64
skin tone, 64–5
slimming pills, 57–9
smoking, 111–22
  and body image, 113–16
  and body weight, 112–13
  cessation, 119–20
  e-cigarettes, 122
  facial ageing and, 116–19

initiation, 120–1
and weight loss, 5–6, 60–2
Social Cognitive Theory, 67–8
Sociocultural Attitudes Towards Appearance Scale-3 (SATAQ-3), 159
sociocultural pressures, drug use and, 19–20
sports environment/participation, drug use and, 21–2
sports performance/appearance, drug and substance use and, 66
sports supplements, advertising of, 93–106
  body dissatisfaction and, 94–6
  body image and, 94–6
  enhancement, 96–8
  enhancement with health, merging, 98–102
  as foretaste of future, 105–6
  as mirror to twenty-first century health, 102–5
steroids
  anabolic, and muscularity, 6
  anabolic-androgenic, 38–43, 55–6
  and muscularity, 14–15
  precursors, and muscularity, 15
stigma, NMUPS for weight loss and, 159–60
substance abuse
  boys, 22–3
  male adolescents, 22–3
Substance Abuse and Mental Health Services Administration (SAMHSA)
  National Survey on Drug Use and Health, 149
sugar-sweetened beverage (SSB), 81–2

suicidal ideation, drug use and, 46
suppressors of cytokine signalling (SOCS), 206
synthol, and muscularity, 6
synthol, bodybuilders use of, 127–43
   credibility, 138–43
   data analysis, 131–2
   data collection, 129–31
   ethics of, 130–1
   legitimation, 133–4
   results, 132
   support, 134–7

T

tanning products, 64–5
tetraiodothyronine (T_4), 213
   for obesity, 177, 184–7
thyroid function, growth hormone effects on, 212–14
thyroid-stimulating hormone (TSH), 213
thyroid system, 185
thyrotropin-releasing hormone (TRH), 213
thyroxine
   replacement therapy, 186
   for weight loss, 5
tobacco
   and weight loss, 15
   See also smoking
topiramate (TPM), for obesity, 192
triiodothyronine (T_3), 213
   for obesity, 177, 184–7

V

video gaming magazines
   exposure to, drug use and, 19–20
"Virginia Slims" campaign, 54, 60

W

weightlifting, and muscle dysmorphia, 36–7
weight loss
   ADHD medications for, off-label use of, 153–5
   using drugs, 5–6
weight status, drug use and, 18
World Anti-Doping Agency (WADA), 202, 205

Y

Yale-Brown Obsessive Compulsive Scale, 18

The manufacturer's authorised representative in the EU is Springer Nature Customer Service Centre GmbH, Europaplatz 3, 69115 Heidelberg, Germany. If you have any concerns regarding our products, please contact ProductSafety@springernature.com

Printed and bound by CPI Group (UK) Ltd, Croydon, CR0 4YY

23/03/2026

02076449-0002